Springer
Tokyo
Berlin
Heidelberg
New York
Barcelona
Budapest
Hong Kong
London
Milan
Paris
Santa Clara
Singapore

H. Ozawa · T. Saito · N. Takahata (Eds.)

Signal Transduction in Affective Disorders

With 40 Figures

Springer

Hiroki Ozawa, M.D., Ph.D.
Instructor, Department of Neuropsychiatry, School of Medicine, Sapporo Medical University, S-1, W-16, Chuo-ku, Sapporo, Hokkaido 060, Japan

Toshikazu Saito, M.D., Ph. D.
Professor, Department of Occupational Therapy, School of Health Science, Sapporo Medical University, S-1, W-16, Chuo-ku, Sapporo, Hokkaido 060, Japan

Naohiko Takahata, M.D., Ph.D.
Professor, Department of Neuropsychiatry, School of Medicine, Sapporo Medical University, S-1, W-16, Chuo-ku, Sapporo, Hokkaido 060, Japan

ISBN 978-4-431-70210-8 Springer-Verlag Tokyo Berlin Heidelberg New York

Library of Congress Cataloging-in-Publication Data

Signal transduction in affective disorders / H. Ozawa, T. Saito, N. Takahata (eds.).
p. cm.
Proceedings of papers presented at the Symposium on Affective Disorders and Neuronal Signal Transduction at the 92nd General Meeting of the Japanese Society of Psychiatry and Neurology in Sapporo, Japan, May 23, 1996 and from the 11th Sapporo Neuroscience Meeting held March 1, 1996.
Includes bibliographical references and index.
ISBN 978-4-431-70210-8 (hardcover : alk. paper)
1. Affective disorders—Pathophysiology—Congresses. 2. Neural transmission—Congresses. 3. Antidepressants—Mechanism of action—Congresses. 4. Cellular signal transduction—Congresses. I. Ozawa, H. (Hiroki), 1960- . II. Saito, Toshikazu. III. Takahata, Naohiko, 1932- . IV. Nihon Seishin Shinkei Gakkai. Sokai (92nd : 1996: Sapporo-shi, Japan) V. Symposium on Affective Disorders and Neuronal Signal Transduction (1996 : Sapporo-shi, Japan) VI. Sapporo Neuroscience Meeting (11th : 1996)
[DNLM: 1. Affective Disorders—physiopathology—congresses. 2. Affective Disorders—drug therapy—congresses. 3. Antidepressive Agents—pharmacology—congresses. 4. Signal Transduction—drug effects—congresses. WM 171 S578 1997]
RC537.S534 1998
616.89'07—dc21
DNLM/DLC
for Library of Congress 97-44757

Printed on acid-free paper

Typesetting: Best-set Typesetter Ltd., Hong Kong

SPIN: 10644636

Preface

Recent progress in brain science has been remarkable, especially with regard to advances in the area of neuroscience. Particularly in the past decade, there have been many important discoveries about signal transduction in the brain. With this background, biological research in affective disorders has become well developed in relation to neural signaling. However, this field is fairly hard to understand comprehensively, and there is relatively little integrative work with clinical psychiatry in spite of the involvement of a wide variety of scientific disciplines.

This monograph brings together up-to-date reviews from several young Japanese scientists who work in basic and clinical neuroscience. The intention is to explain in plain language the information that has evolved on signal transduction in terms of the biological abnormalities and mechanisms of antidepressants. The model shown on the cover (and on page 24) is intended to help the reader understand signal transduction in the brain and the pathophysiology of affective disorders as well as the mechanisms of antidepressants.

The book proceeds in the order presented in this model. T. Saito begins with a comprehensive review of the neural signal transduction system and of critical issues in previous hypotheses on affective disorders and the mechanisms of antidepressants. O. Tajima and colleagues address the topic of serotonin and noradrenergic neuromodulation of pre- and post-synapses in the hippocampus using in vivo microdialysis and intracellular recording to examine the net effects of chronic antidepressant treatments in rats. The chapter by I. Kusumi and T. Koyama focuses on neuroendocrine studies of the dysregulation of $5HT_{2A}$ receptor functions in affective disorders as well as peripheral tissue studies on the enhancement of 5HT-induced calcium mobilization in platelets in affective disorders. Writing about the background of calcium signaling abnormalities in affective disorders, A. Kagaya and S. Yamawaki describe the integration of immune function and intracellular calcium signaling in terms of the pathophysiology of mood disorders.

Chapters 5–7 concentrate on cAMP-related signal pathways connected to the pathophysiology of affective disorders and the action mechanisms of antidepressants. Through postmortem examination of the human brain, H. Ozawa and N. Takahata discuss the imbalance of G protein functions in affective disorders and its relation to the action of antidepressants. S. Miyamoto and M. Asakura focus on the cAMP-dependent phosphorylation system of microtubulin after administration of antidepressants. S. Morinobu and colleagues address the further-downstream cAMP signaling pathway related to a neurotrophic factor (BDNF) and neuroplasticity in stress-related psychiatric disorders. Additionally, Y. Odagaki and colleagues provide an overview of reports dealing with the effects of lithium, focusing on the respective components of postreceptor signal transduction systems mediated through G protein-coupled receptors. S. Hatta and H. Ohshika address the role of cytoskeletal components (tubulin) in signal transduction involving the action of antidepressants. Finally, T. Kato discusses the possibilities of applying magnetic resonance spectroscopy (MRS) in in vivo investigations of signal transduction systems in affective disorders.

The editors appreciate the contributions received from investigators who are active in the field. This volume presents papers from the Symposium on Affective Disorders and Neuronal Signal Transduction, chaired by Prof. T. Higuchi and Prof. T. Saito at the 92nd General Meeting of the Japanese Society of Psychiatry and Neurology (Prof. N. Takahata, President) in Sapporo, Japan, May 23, 1996, and from the 11th Sapporo Neuroscience Meeting in Sapporo, Japan, March 1, 1996.

This publication was financially supported in part by a grant-in-aid (No. 97010) for publication of scientific research results from the Ministry of Education, Science, Sports and Culture of Japan and by the Ministry of Health and Welfare.

Finally, we would like to thank the staff of Springer-Verlag Tokyo for their patience and encouragement.

T. Higuchi
N. Takahata
June 1997

Contents

Effects of Antidepressants on Transmembrane Signaling

Toshikazu Saito

Introduction

Antidepressants are widely used for depression and other psychiatric disorders, but their neurochemical mechanism of action is still unclear. The monoamine hypothesis of affective disorders (Schildkraut 1965) proposes that antidepressants exhibit their therapeutic effects by inhibition of monoamine reuptake in presynaptic nerve terminals, which leads to facilitation of monoamine transmission. However, the acute effects of antidepressants on neurotransmission are inconsistent with the delayed onset of their clinical efficacy (Zelman and Garver 1990). Moreover, some monoamine reuptake inhibitors, such as cocaine, do have not an antidepressant effect.

Vetulani and Sulser (1975) demonstrated that chronic antidepressant administration results in a reduction of the number of β-adrenergic receptors in rats. This receptor down-regulation occurs with a delayed response but before the development of clinical therapeutic effects. Selective serotonin reuptake inhibitors (SSRIs) have little effect on β-receptors but do have an antidepressive effect similar to that of tricyclic antidepressants. Moreover, chronic tricyclic antidepressant administration is reported to cause a reduction of serotonin receptors (Peroutka and Snyder 1980), though there does not appear to be consistent alteration of serotonin-2 receptors by SSRIs.

These results suggest that the receptor changes caused by tricyclic antidepressants may not be related to the antidepressive effect or may only be involved in the first step of the cascade of signal transduction involved in it. Therefore, recent studies searching for a common mechanism of antidepressant action have focused on postreceptor neuronal cell signaling processes as potential targets of such action (Menkes et al. 1983; Ozawa and Rasenick 1989).

Department of Occupational Therapy, School of Health Sciences, Sapporo Medical University, S.3, W.17, Chuo-ku, Sapporo, Hokkaido 060, Japan

Role of G Proteins in Signal Transduction

β-Receptors and serotonin receptors are linked to the adenylyl cyclase or phospholipase C system. G proteins, which have a common heterotrimeric structure consisting of α, β, and γ subunits, play an important role in signal transduction in these systems, wherein agonist interaction with receptors promotes the formation of a ternary agonist–receptor–G protein complex. In this complex, G protein is bound to guanosine diphosphate (GDP). The agonist binding facilitates the change from GDP into guanosine triphosphate (GTP). When GTP binds to the α subunit, the receptor–G protein complex dissociates. This results in release of the receptor and the α subunit from the β and γ subunits of G protein, which can also act as signal transducers. The GTP-bound form of the α subunit is the active form of this protein, which can activate the catalytic subunit of the enzyme. The α subunit of G protein shuts itself off by hydrolyzing the bound GTP to GDP via intrinsic GTPases. Following this action, the agonist stimulation of the system can be repeated. In the adenylyl cyclase system, G_s and G_i proteins regulate stimulation and inhibition of adenylyl cyclase, thereby altering the concentration of the intracellular mediator cyclic AMP (Gilman 1987; Birnbaumer 1990).

In the phospholipase C system, G_q protein activates phosphoinositide-specific phospholipase C (phospholipase C-β). This in turn hydrolyzes phosphatidylinositol bisphosphate (PIP_2) to inositol 1,4,5-trisphosphate (IP_3), which increases the intracellular level of Ca^{2+} by releasing Ca^{2+} from the endoplasmic reticulum, and that of diacylglycerol, which remains in the membrane and activates protein kinase C (C-kinase) (Sekar and Hokin 1986; Asaoka et al. 1992; Harden 1992).

Increases in the levels of intracellular cyclic AMP and Ca^{2+} cause activation of cyclic AMP-dependent protein kinase (A-kinase) and Ca/calmodulin-dependent protein kinase (CaM-kinase), respectively. These kinases alter the activities of target proteins by phosphorylation, thereby inducing alterations of cell signaling (Cohen 1988; Walaas and Greengard 1991; Asaoka et al. 1992). It has been reported that A-kinase and C-kinase can activate the transcription of specific genes via protein phosphorylation. C-kinase, for example, activates a phosphorylation cascade that leads to the phosphorylation and activation of a mitogen-activated protein (MAP) kinase. The activated MAP kinase regulates transcription by phosphorylation and activation of the DNA-bound generegulatory protein Elk-1 (Hunter and Karin 1992).

A-kinase phosphorylates and activates cyclic AMP response element-binding protein (CREB). This activated CREB then turns on gene transcription via binding of cyclic AMP response element (CRE) sites located in the promoter regions of genes. CREB is also phosphorylated and activated by CaM-kinase and C-kinase (Brindle and Montminy 1992). Brain-derived neurotrophic factor (BDNF), a nerve growth factor, reportedly supports the differentiation and survival of neurons, and chronic administration of phosphodiesterase inhibitor increases the expression of BDNF as well as that of CREB (Nibuya et al. 1996). Therefore, it is likely that the cellular cyclic AMP level may be related to the expression of BDNF mRNA.

Effects of Chronic Administration of Antidepressants on Signal Transduction

Our laboratory and others have reported that chronic treatment of rats with tricyclic antidepressants results in an increase guanine nucleotide-stimulated adenylyl cyclase activity by facilitation of G_s function without altering the content of G_s or other G proteins in rat brain membrane (Ozawa and Rasenick 1989; Ozawa et al. 1994). More recently, we observed that chronic SSRI treatment also results in an increase in guanine nucleotide-stimulated adenylyl cyclase activity associated with facilitation of G_s function in rat cerebral cortical membrane (Saito 1997). This antidepressant effect on the adenylyl cyclase system requires 2 to 3 weeks to develop, which correlates well with the time course of the clinical therapeutic response. Furthermore, rolipram, which inhibits phosphodiesterase IV and subsequently increases the cellular cyclic AMP content, also has an antidepressant effect (Bobon et al. 1988). Additionally, hyperfunction of G_i was recently recognized in the cerebral cortex in the postmortem brains of patients with depression (Ozawa et al. 1997). Thus, these findings suggest it is possible that the pharmacological effects of antidepressants occur as a result of normalization of the functional dysbalance between G_s and G_i in the brain. An increase in the level of cyclic AMP leads to activation of A-kinase, which phosphorylates target proteins and thereby causes alterations of cell signaling. This can be seen by the fact that chronic antidepressant treatment elicits changes in the endogenous phosphorylation of MAP-2 in soluble and crude microtubule fractions by A-kinase as well as other protein kinases (Perez et al. 1989; Miyamoto et al. 1995).

Recently, it has been reported that chronic antidepressant treatment inhibits the polymerization of tubulin and increases tubulin dimers in cerebral cortex (Miyamoto et al. 1995). These tubulin dimers activate trimeric G protein function via GTP transfer from tubulin to G proteins (Kamata et al. 1996; Saito 1997). It has also been suggested that chronic antidepressant treatment stimulates the translocation of A-kinase downstream in the cyclic AMP pathway (Nestler et al. 1989). Furthermore, long-term treatment with antidepressants, including SSRIs, brings about a significant increase in CREB mRNA in rat hippocampus (Nibuya et al. 1996). Taken together, the above findings strongly suggest that the cyclic AMP-A kinase-gene expression cascade is a common target of various types of antidepressants and that changes in the cascade induced by chronic antidepressant treatment may be related to the late onset of clinical efficacy of these drugs.

The Phospholipase C System in Affective Disorders

Other studies have indicated that alterations in the phospholipase C system are important in the pathophysiology of affective disorders. Stimulation of 5-HT receptors has been indicated to increase phosphoinositide hydrolysis in human platelets (De Chaffoy de Courcelles et al. 1985). This results in production of IP_3, which increases the intracellular level of Ca^{2+} by releasing it from internal storage sites. Recent studies have reported that 5-HT-induced Ca^{2+} mobilization is enhanced in the platelets of unmedicated patients with major depression (Koyama et al. 1993; Yamawaki et al. 1996). Moreover, Walden et al. (1995) have demonstrated that Ca^{2+}-channel antagonists have a clinical effect when used for treatment of affective disorders. On the other hand, Pandey et al. (1991) demonstrated that antidepressant treatment in vitro increased levels of phosphatidylinositol (PI), PI-4-phosphate (PIP), and PI 4,5-bisphosphate (PIP_2) in both human platelets and rat cerebral cortex. Based on these results, they suggested that antidepressant treatment inhibits phospholipase C activity. Thus, it is possible that up-regulation of the phospholipase C system may occur in patients with depressive disorders and the clinical efficacy of these drugs may be due to the fact that they normalize the system. However, the relationship between the effects of antidepressants on the phospholipase C system and their clinical efficacy is still unclear.

Targets for Antidepressants

The observations reported in the studies reviewed above suggest that multiple neural dysfunctions may exist in patients with depressive disorders and that there are, therefore, multiple targets for antidepressants. Wachtel (1990) proposed the second-messenger dysbalance hypothesis of affective disorders. According to this theory, affective disorders are caused by a functional imbalance of the two major intraneural signal-amplification systems, with depression resulting from hypofunction of the adenylyl cyclase system together with absolute or relative dominance of the phospholipase C system. Although most findings of the studies reviewed above appear to be consistent with the second-messenger dysbalance hypothesis, further studies are required to determine the exact nature of neurochemical dysfunctions of depressive disorders and the actions of antidepressants on the second messenger–protein kinase–gene expression cascade, which may be related to long-term adaptive or plastic changes in the molecular mechanisms of these drugs. Moreover, progress in research on cell signaling in depressive disorders may lead to new insights, resulting in the development of new and novel antidepressants.

References

Asaoka Y, Nakamura S-I, Yoshida K, Nishizuka Y (1992) Protein kinase C, calcium and phospholipid degradation. Trends Biochem Sci 17:414–417

Birnbaumer L (1990) G protein in signal transduction. Annu Rev Pharmacol Toxicol 30:675–705

Bobon D, Breulet M, Gerard-Vandenhove MA, Guiot-Goffioul F, Plomteux G, Sastre y Hernandez M, Troisfontaines B, von Frenckell R, Wachtel H (1988) Is phosphodiesterase inhibition a new mechanism of antidepressant action? A double blind double-dummy study between rolipram and desipramine in hospitalized major and/or endogenous depressives. Eur Arch Psychiatry Neurol Sci 238:2–6

Brindle PK, Montminy MR (1992) The CREB family of transcription activators. Curr Opin Gen Dev 2:119–204

Cohen P (1988) Protein phosphorylation and hormone action. Proc R Soc Lond (Biol) 234:115–144

De Chaffy de Courcelles D, Leysen JE, De Clerck F, Van Belle H, Janssen PA (1985) Evidence that phospholipid turnover is the signal transducing system coupled to serotonin-S2 receptor sites. J Biol Chem 260:7603–7608

Gilman AG (1987) G proteins: transducers of receptor-generated signals. Annu Rev Biochem 56:615–649

Harden TK (1992) G-protein-regulated phospholipase C: identification of component proteins. Adv Second Messenger Phosphoprotein Res 26:225–250

Hunter T, Karin M (1992) The regulation of transcription by phosphorylation. Cell 70:375–387

Kamata H, Ozawa H, Saito T, Hatta H, Takahata N(1996) Dimeric tubulin stimulated adenylyl cyclase activity after long-term amitriptyline treatment. Life Sci 60:57–66

Koyama T, Kusumi I, Matsubara S, Yamashita I (1993) Study on biological markers in serotonergic system of affective disorders-Significance of serotonin2 receptor function in the pathophysiology of depression. Annual Report of the National Project Team of Biological Studies on Pathogenesis and Treatment of Affective Disorders, Ministry of Health and Welfare, Japan, pp 71–76

Menkes DB, Rasenick MM, Wheeler MA, Bitensky M (1983) Guanosine triphosphate activation of brain adenylate cyclase: enhancement by long term antidepressant treatment. Science 219:65–67

Miyamoto S, Asakura M, Sasuga Y (1995) Effects of chronic administration of antidepressants on microtubule assembly in rat cerebral cortex. Jpn J Psychopharmacol 15:385–395

Nestler EJ, Terwilliger RZ, Duman RS (1989) Chronic antidepressant administration alters the subcellular distribution of cyclic AMP-dependent protein kinase in rat frontal cortex. J Neurochem 53:1644–1647

Nibuya M, Nestler EJ, Duman RS (1996) Chronic antidepressant administration increases the expression of cyclic AMP response element binding protein (CREB) in rat hyppocampus. J Neurosci 16:2365–2372

Ozawa H, Rasenick MM (1989) Coupling of the stimulatory GTP-binding protein Gs to rat synaptic membrane adenylate cyclase is enhanced subsequent to chronic antidepressant treatment. Mol Pharmacol 36:803–808

Ozawa H, Katamura Y, Hatta S, Amemiya N, Saito T, Ohshika H, Takahata N (1994) Antidepressants directly influence in situ binding of guanine nucleotide in synaptic membrane. Life Sci 54:925–932

Ozawa H, Hashimoto E, Saito T, Yamamoto M, Maeda H, Takahata N, Gsell W, Frolich L, Riederer P (1997) Cyclic AMP production and degradation systems in postmortem cortex of depressed patients. J Neural Transmi (Gen Sec) in press

Pandey GN, Pandey SC, Davis JM (1991) Effect of desipramine on inositol phosphate formation and inositol phospholipids in rat brain and human platelets. Psychopharmacol Bull 27:255–261
Perez J, Tinelli D, Brunello N, Racagni G (1989) cAMP-dependent phosphorylation of soluble and crude microtuble fractions of rat cerebral cortex after prolonged desmethylimipramine treatment. Eur J Pharmacol Sec 172:305–316
Peroutka SJ, Snyder SH (1980) Long-term antidepressant tratment decreases spiroperidol-labeled serotonin receptor binding. Science 210:88–90
Saito T (1997) Changes in G protein-mediated signal transduction in affective disorders. Jpn J Neuropsychophatmacol 19:83–90
Schildkraut JJ (1965) The catecholamine hypothesis of affective disorders; a review of supporting evidence. Am J Psychiatry 122:509–520
Sekar MC, Hokin LE (1965) The role of phosphoinositides in signal transduction. J Membr Biol 89:193–210
Vetulani J, Sulser F (1975) Action of various antidepressant treatments reduces reactivity of noradrenergic cyclic AMP-generating system in limbic forebrain. Nature 257:495–496
Wachtel H (1990) The second-messenger dysbalance hypothesis of affective disorders. Pharmacopsychiatry 23:27–32
Walass SI, Greengard P (1991) Protein phosphorylation and neuronal function. Pharmacol Rev 43:299–349
Walden J, Fritze J, Van Calker D, Berger M, Grunze H (1995) A calcium antagonist for the treatment of depressive episodes: singlecase reports. J Psychiatr Res 29:71–76
Yamawaki S, Kagaya A, Okamoto Y, Uchitomi Y, Shimizu M, Nishida A (1996) Role of intracellular calcium mechanisms in the pathophysiology of affective disorders. In: Shibuya T (ed) International Academy for Biomedical and Drug Research. Vol. 11. Preclinical and clinical strategies for the treatment of neurodegenerative, cerebrovascular and mental disorders. Karger, Basel, pp 106-115
Zelman FP, Garver DL (1990) Depression and antidepressant therapy: receptor dynamics. Prog Neuropsychopharmacol Biol Psychiatry 14:503–523

Serotonergic and Noradrenergic Neuromodulation in the Hippocampus and the Mechanism of Action of Antidepressants

Osamu Tajima, Shinichi Murata, Tsukasa Mitsuhashi, and Kenichi Takemasa

Introduction

Despite the recent explosive progress of brain imaging and molecular biology, the pathophysiology of affective disorders and the mechanism of action of antidepressant drugs remain unknown. There is no consensus about the net effect of chronic antidepressant treatment on serotonergic and noradrenergic neurotransmission, particularly noradrenergic neurotransmission. Novel antidepressants, such as selective serotonin (5-HT) reuptake inhibitors (SSRIs) or reversible inhibitors of monoamine oxidase A (RIMAs) have better side-effect profiles and wide clinical indications compared with classical tricyclic antidepressants. SSRIs such as fluoxetine, sertraline, fluvoxamine, paroxetine, and citalopram have little anticholinergic effect and have been proved to be effective not only for depression but also for obsessive-compulsive disorder, panic disorder, and eating disorder. RIMAs do not have the fatal side effect of old irreversible monoamine oxidase inhibitors, the so-called cheese effect, and among RIMAs such as moclobemide, brofaramine, and toloxatone, moclobemide has efficacy against social phobia. The clinical efficacy of these novel antidepressants against major depression, however, is not significantly different from that of classical antidepressants. The clinical choice of an antidepressant for an individual patient remains primarily based on considerations of side effects and safety rather than efficacy (Lecrubier 1993).

Therefore, to elucidate the biological basis of affective disorders and the mechanism of action of antidepressants, we have investigated the biological markers for affective disorders and the mechanism of action of antidepressants in animal studies; the plasma levels of 3-methoxy-4-hydroxyphenylglycol

Kyorin University School of Medicine, Department of Neuropsychiatry, 6-20-2, Shinkawa, Mitaka, Tokyo 181, Japan

(MHPG), a major metabolite of noradrenaline, in patients with major depression before and during antidepressant treatment; cerebral blood flow in the acute phase and during remission using N-isopropyl-p-I-123-iodoamphetamine (I-123-IMP) single-photon emission computerized tomography (SPECT); the effects of acute and chronic administration of various antidepressants on the firing activity of locus coeruleus noradrenergic neurons; the effects of forced swimming on monoamine metabolism in vivo and the effects of antidepressants on forced swimming-induced changes in monoamine metabolism; and the effects of antidepressants on the excitability of hippocampal pyramidal cells and their intracellular signal-transduction systems.

The hippocampus may play an important role in learning, memory, and epileptic seizures. Long-term potentiation in the hippocampus and long-term depression in the cerebellum are well-known examples of neural plasticity in the central nervous system (CNS). Recent studies using functional magnetic resonance imaging (MRI) indicate that the hippocampus may be responsible for episodic memory. The hippocampus receives monoaminergic projections from the brain stem. Corticotropin-releasing factor (CRF) receptors are abundant in the hippocampus. Recent studies suggest a close association of the hippocampus with anxiety disorders and stress disorders. The common mechanism of almost all known antidepressants is related to potentiation of central monoaminergic transmission. Most postsynaptic monoamine receptors except the 5-HT_3 receptor, which is directly coupled to an ion channel, couple with guanine nucleotide-binding protein (G protein), which regulates the intracellular signal transduction systems such as cyclic AMP (Gilman 1987; Birnbaumer 1990).

Classical neurotransmitters such as 5-HT, noradrenaline, and dopamine may play a role as neruomodulators in the CNS that regulate the neuronal excitability of the postsynaptic neurons (Madison and Nicoll 1982; Andrade and Nicoll 1987; McCormick et al. 1991; Kohler et al. 1996). Synchronous changes in neuronal excitability in the cerebral cortex, which receives monosynaptic aminergic projections from the locus coeruleus, or the raphe of the brain stem after chronic antidepressant treatment might be closely related to the mechanism of action of antidepressants. In this chapter we present our pathophysiological model of affective disorders and examine the novel antidepressants in terms of their pharmacological characteristics in order to elucidate whether a final common pathway of antidepressant action exists. We then describe our studies using in vivo microdialysis and intracellular recording that examine the net effects of the repeated administration of antidepressants on monoaminergic neuromodulation in the hippocampus. Finally, we discuss which neuronal plastic changes after chronic antidepressant treatment may be involved in the mechanism of action of these drugs from the neurodynamic point of view (Cohen and Servan-Schreiber 1993) and suggest future directions of research.

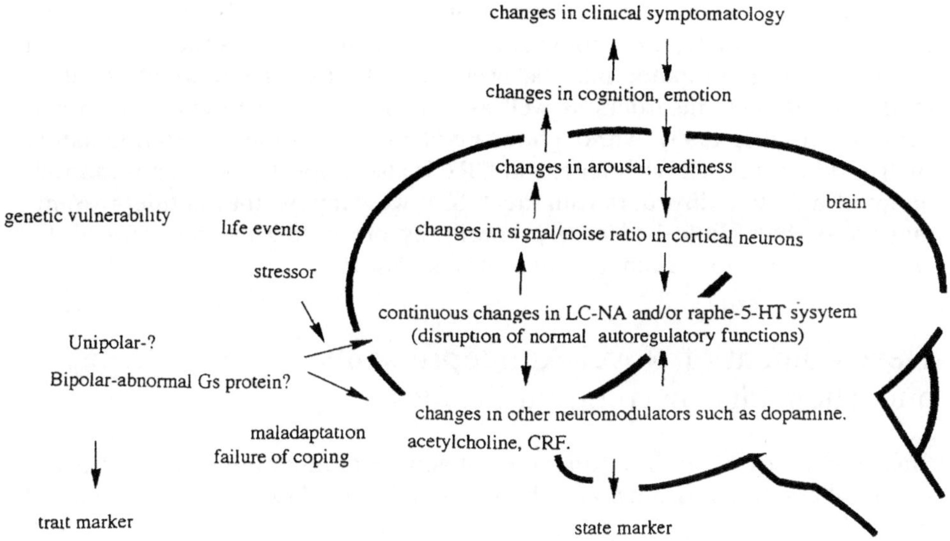

FIG. 1. Monoaminergic modulation of information processing in the brain and the vulnerability-stress model of affective disorders. *5-HT*, serotomin; *LC*, locus coeruleus; *NA*, noradrenaline; *CRF*, corticotropin releasing factor

Pathophysiological Model of Affective Disorders and Monoaminergic Function

Figure 1 shows our pathophysiological model of affective disorders. The model suggests that abnormalities in G proteins, which transduce and amplify the signals from receptors to intracellular second-messenger systems, may be involved in bipolar disorder. Particularly, abnormally increased activities are demonstrated in Gs proteins, which activate adenylate cyclase, which then produces cyclic AMP, one of the most important intracellular second messengers. Many studies suggest that unipolar depression may be a heterogeneous group of disorders. Stressful life events, especially object loss and failure of coping behavior, such as overadaptation, may be involved in triggering unipolar depression.

Acute stress may stimulate central noradrenergic and serotonergic activities. We suspect that chronic stress may disrupt the autoregulatory functions in the central monoaminergic nervous systems that decrease the signal/noise (S/N) ratio. Modulation of the S/N ratio in cortical neurons seems to be a common neurophysiological function in the central noradrenergic and serotonergic nervous systems. A decrease in the S/N ratio in the cortex means a decrease in vigilance and readiness of the organism (McCormick et al. 1991). Although we do not know the exact relationships between the changes in information processing in the cerebral cortex and the clinical symptomatology of affective disorders, a neurodynamic model that simulates the information processing in a computer may be useful for discussing the comprehensive model of affective disorders as well as schizophrenic disorders (Cohen and Servan-Schreiber 1993). Although the involvement of other neuromodulators such as dopamine, acetylcholine, and CRF is also suspected in the pathophysiology of affective disorders (Sugrue 1983), we suppose that antidepressants may exert their clinical efficacy primarily by promoting the recovery of decreased central monoaminergic neurotransmission.

Development of Novel Antidepressants and Their Pharmacological Profiles

Since the discovery of the antidepressant actions of imipramine, the prototype of tricyclic antidepressants, and the monoamine oxidase inhibitor iproniazid more than four decades ago, a variety of novel antidepressant drugs with different pharmacological properties have been developed. Among these novel antidepressants, SSRIs such as fluoxetine, fluvoxamine, sertraline, and citalopram are widely used for the treatment not only of depression but also of panic disorder, obsessive-compulsive disorder, and eating disorder. Another class of antidepressants consists of dual (NA and 5-HT) reuptake inhibitors with minimal additional receptor activities, such as venlafaxine, milnacipran, and duloxetine (Fig. 2). Despite the enormous efforts to discover more effective and faster-acting drugs, almost all known antidepressants exert their

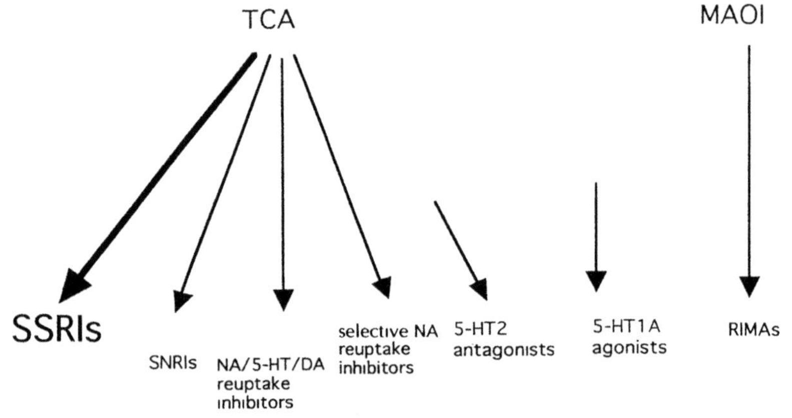

Fig. 2. Development of novel antidepressants and their pharmacologic properties. *DA*, dopamine; *MAOI*, monoamine oxidase inhibitor; *NA*, noradrenaline; *SSRIs*, selective serotonin reuptake inhibitors; *RIMAs*, reversible inhibitors of monoamine oxidase A; *TCA*, tricyclic antidepressant; *SNRIs*, serotonin/noradrenaline reuptake inhibitors

clinical efficacy through monoaminergic neurotransmission, and there are no significant differences in clinical efficacy between the novel antidepressants, such as SSRIs, and the old tricyclics (Lecrubier 1993; Brunello et al. 1994/1995; Kasper et al. 1994/1995).

Modulation of Serotonergic Neurotransmission by SSRIs

Although a variety of pharmacologically different antidepressants are now available, the mainstay of the pharmacological treatment of depressive disorders is still the inhibitors of serotonin and/or noradrenaline reuptake. Recently, the structures of the monoamine transporters in the presynaptic nerve terminals that are target proteins of monoamine reuptake inhibitors have been determined by molecular biological techniques (Blakely et al. 1991; Hoffman et al. 1991; Pacholczyk et al. 1991), but we still do not know the exact mechanism of action of antidepressants. Since the discovery of the down-regulation of β-adrenergic receptors after chronic treatment with pharmacologically different antidepressants and electroconvulsive shock (Sulser 1984), contradictory hypotheses have been proposed, and we have no consensus about the net effects of repeated treatment with antidepressants on central noradrenergic neurotransmission. Some researchers have indicated a net decrease, and others have suggested a net increase, in monoaminergic neurotransmission after chronic antidepressant treatment. In contrast, recent biochemical and electrophysiological studies on the net effects of chronic antidepressant treatment on central serotonergic neurotransmission have consistently demonstrated a net increase in serotonergic neurotransmission (Blier et al. 1990; Chaput et al. 1991). Biochemical studies using in vivo brain dialysis showed that SSRIs significantly increased the extracellular level of 5-HT in the frontal cortex, hypothalamus, and hippocampus. Electrophysiological investigations clearly indicated that long-term administration of tricyclic antidepressants enhanced 5-HT neurotransmission by increasing the responsiveness of postsynaptic neurons to microiontophoretically applied 5-HT through 5-HT_{1A} receptors (De Montigny and Aghajanian 1978). In contrast to tricyclics, SSRIs and monoamine oxidase inhibitors (MAOIs) produce the same net effect by enhancing the function of 5-HT, producing a desensitization of somatodendritic and terminal 5-HT_{1A} autoreceptors and thus reducing their inhibitory effect on the firing activity of 5-HT neurons and on the release of 5-HT, respectively (De Montigny et al. 1991).

We investigated the effects of chronic administration of fluvoxamine on 5-HT levels in the hippocampus using in vivo brain microdialysis. It is clearly suggested that changes in the amount of 5-HT in dialysate collected from semipermeable dialysis membranes inserted in the discrete brain area may reflect changes in the amount of 5-HT released into the synaptic cleft. The levels of 5-HT and dopamine in dialysate collected through a semipermeable dialysis probe from the hippocampus of a freely moving rat were measured by

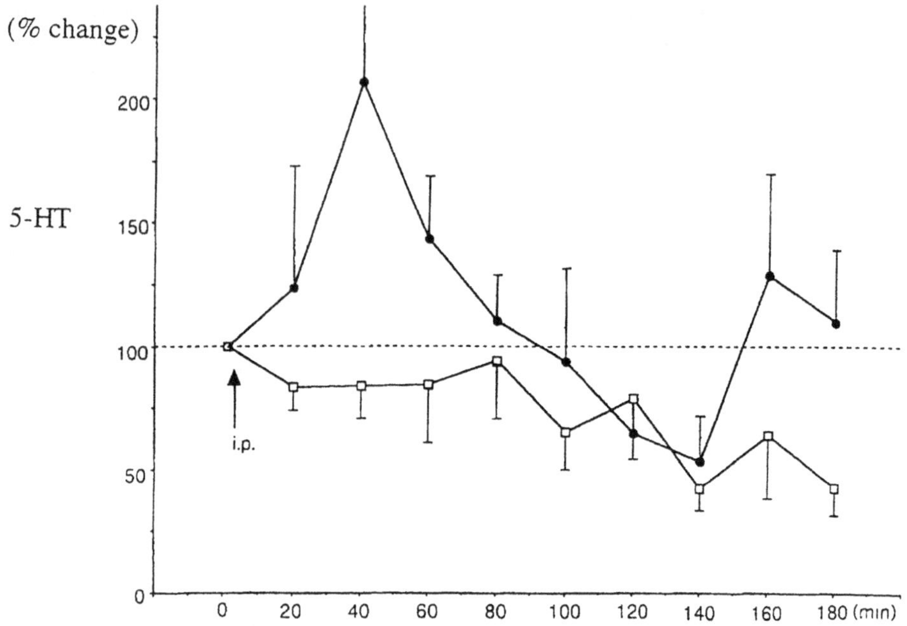

FIG. 3. In vivo changes of 5-HT in dialysate collected from the rat hippocampus following single i.p. administration of 60 mg/kg fluvoxamine (*solid circles*) as saline (*open squares*) ANOVA

on-line high-performance liquid chromatography with electrochemical detection. Figures. 3 and 4 show the changes in 5-HT levels after acute and chronic fluvoxamine administration, respectively.

Figure 3 shows a significant increase in 5-HT in the dialysate collected from the hippocampus of a male Wistar rat after a single intraperitoneal injection of 60 mg/kg fluvoxamine. In contrast to the transient increase in 5-HT after a single administration of fluvoxamine, chronic pretreatment with 10 mg/kg /day fluvoxamine subcutaneously with an osmotic minipump for 14 days significantly enhanced the effect of an additional i.p. administration of fluvoxamine of the same dose 60 mg/kg on 5-HT in dialysate from the hippocampus, compared with that in saline controls (Fig. 4). Down-regulation of terminal and somatodendritic 5-HT autoreceptors may be involved in the enhancement of the 5-HT response after chronic fluvoxamine treatment. It is clearly shown that acute administration of tricyclic antidepressants strongly inhibited the firing activity of noradrenergic and serotonergic neurons in proportion to the potency of their inhibition of monoamine reuptake (Scuvee-Moreau and Dresse 1979). In contrast, chronic administration of tricyclic antidepressants significantly attenuated the inhibitory action of these drugs, reflecting the down-regulation of somatodendritic α_2 autoreceptors. Thus, contrary to the earlier suggestion that the increase in 5-HT and/or noradrenaline in the synap-

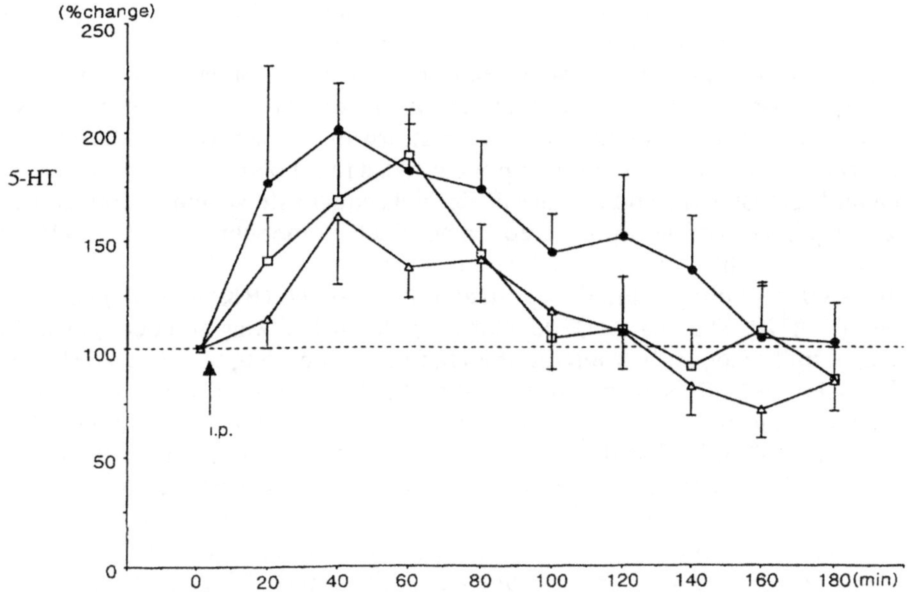

FIG. 4. Effects of chronic fluvoxamine pretreatment on 5-HT in the rat hippocampus. After chronic fluvoxamine treatment, 10 mg/kg/day for 14 days by an osmotic minipump implanted in the dorsal subcutaneous tissue of the rat, an additional i.p. injection of fluvoxamine at 60 mg/kg (*solid circles*) as 30 mg/kg (*open squares*) was administered. *Open triangle* show response to an i.p. injection of 60 mg/kg fluvoxamine after IH days of pretreatment with saline ANOVA

tic cleft may appear soon after a single dose of monoamine reuptake inhibitor, a continuous increase in synaptic monoamine may appear only after chronic administration of these drugs until down-regulation of the autoreceptors occurs.

Convergence of Serotonergic and Noradrenergic Neurotransmission: Neurodynamic Viewpoint

It is suggested that plastic changes in neurons after repeated administration of antidepressants may be related to the mechanism of antidepressant action. Although the recent explosive progress in molecular biological techniques is expected to elucidate the exact mechanism of action of antidepressants, it is necessary to integrate the molecular level into the neurophysiological and cognitive levels to explain the exact mechanism of action. Therefore we investigated the electrophysiological action of antidepressants, with special reference to the physiological function of the central monoaminergic systems, because most of the previous studies did not consider the physiological function of the central serotonergic and noradrenergic systems.

The action potential in the vertebrate neuron is followed by an afterhyperpolarization (AHP) that may persist for several seconds and may have profound consequences for the firing pattern of the neuron. The AHP has several components. The fast component helps to repolarize the action potential and regulates the spike interval. The subsequent slow components underlie adaptation of the spike frequency. Each component of the AHP is mediated by different Ca^{2+}-activated K^+ channels. The large-conductance (100–200 pS), voltage- and Ca^{2+}-activated K^+ channels (BK channels) underlie the fast AHP. The fast AHP develops rapidly in 1 to 2 ms and decays within tens of milliseconds. In contrast, the channels underlying the slow AHP (SK channels) are more sensitive to Ca^{2+} than the BK channels, are activated in a voltage-insensitive manner, and have a smaller unit conductance than the BK channels (5–20 pS). The slow AHP varies considerably in different cell types. It is activated, in 10 to 1000 ms, and may decay over several seconds.

In contrast to the fast AHP, which is blocked by low concentrations of the BK channel blockers tetraethylammonium (TEA) and charybdotoxin, the slow AHP is insensitive to these agents. Activation of SK channels underlies the slow AHP in central neurons. The slow AHP in many neurons is blocked by picomolar concentrations of apamin, a venom toxin. In some cells, such as hippocampal pyramidal neurons, the slow AHP is regulated by transmitters, including both noradrenaline and serotonin, that act through protein kinase. Thus, the SK channels make up a subfamily of Ca^{2+}-activated K^+ channels that play key physiological roles in many cell types, including neurons (Kohler et al. 1996).

Using conventional intracellular recording techniques, we have studied the effects of serotonin and noradrenaline on the slow AHP elicited in the rat hippocampal slice preparation. Consistent with earlier reports, noradrenaline added to the superfusion medium significantly inhibited the slow AHP. The inhibitory effect of noradrenaline on the slow AHP was reversible, because washout with normal medium clearly reversed the effect of noradrenaline. This inhibition of the slow AHP means an increase in the excitability of the pyramidal neurons.

In contrast, 5-HT had more complex effects on the excitability of pyramidal neurons. 5-HT added to the superfusion medium had a biphasic effect—an initial hyperpolarizing effect that means a decrease in the excitability and a delayed inhibition of the slow AHP that means an increase in the excitability of the pyramidal neurons. These results are consistent with the findings of most previous studies using hippocampal slice preparations (Andrade and Nicoll 1987; Madison and Nicoll 1982).

Figures 5 and 6 show the results of studies by Nicoll et al. (Madison and Nicoll 1982; Andrade and Nicoll 1987), who have intensively studied the effects of monoamine on the slow AHP and spike frequency accommodation in rat hippocampal neurons. We have investigated the effects of pharma-

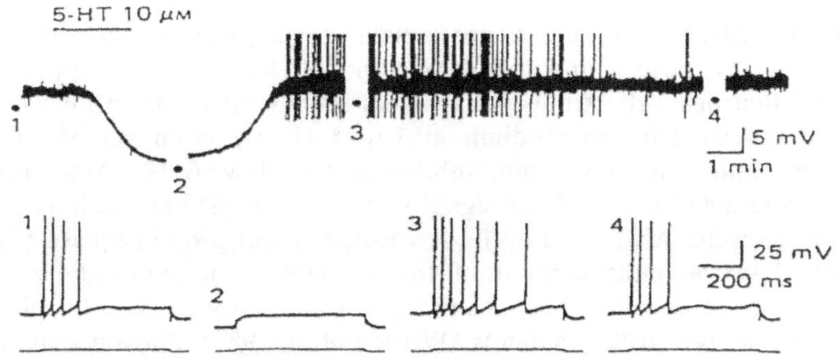

FIG. 5. Effects of 5-HT added to the superfusion medium on the electrophysiological activity of a single pyramidal neuron of the rat hippocampus recorded in vitro (from Andrade and Nicoll 1987 with permission)

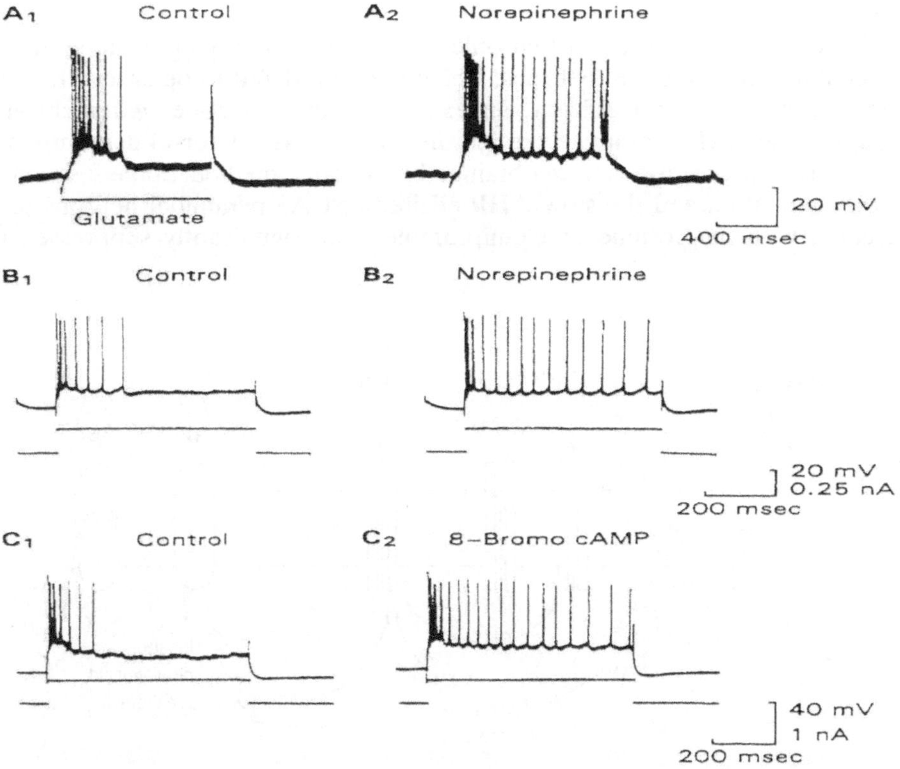

FIG. 6. Effects of norepinephrine and 8-bromo cyclic AMP, a cyclic AMP analogue, on spike frequency accommodation and slow afterhyperpolarization in the CA1 pyramidal neuron recorded in vitro (from Madison and Nicoll 1982 with permission)

cologically different antidepressants, such as maprotiline, clomipramine, fluvoxamine, trazodone, and mianserin, on the slow AHP in hippocampal pyramidal neurons. All of these pharmacologically different antidepressants added to the superfusion medium at 10μM clearly mimicked the effects of noradrenaline and serotonin, inhibiting the slow AHP. Activation of Gs protein-coupled intracellular signal transduction systems, such as adenylate cyclase, cyclic AMP, and cyclic AMP-dependent protein kinase (PKA), is involved in the enhancement of the excitability of pyramidal neurons by noradrenaline and varieties of antidepressants, through the phosphorylation of Ca^{2+}-activated K^+ channels (Worley et al. 1987). Phosphorylation of these particular channels may inhibit the efflux of K^+ from the intracellular cytoplasmic space to the extracellular space, which then leads to the enhancement of excitability. The Ca^{2+}-activated K^+ channels (SK channels) are considered to play a key role in the physiological function of excitable cells, including neurons (Köhler et al. 1996). Protein kinase C (PKC), another important protein kinase in cells, also may inhibit the slow AHP elicited in the hippocampal pyramidal neurons via phosphorylation of the SK channels (Fig. 7).

To elucidate the effects of chronic treatment with antidepressants on the excitability of pyramidal neurons, which are considered to be crucial for the emergence of clinical efficacy, an ex vivo study was done. After chronic maprotiline or clomipramine pretreatment at 5mg/kg i.p. for 14 days, hippocampal slice preparations were obtained by the same method. Spike frequency accommodation and the slow AHP elicited in CA3 pyramidal neurons pretreated with maprotiline or clomipramine were significantly suppressed in

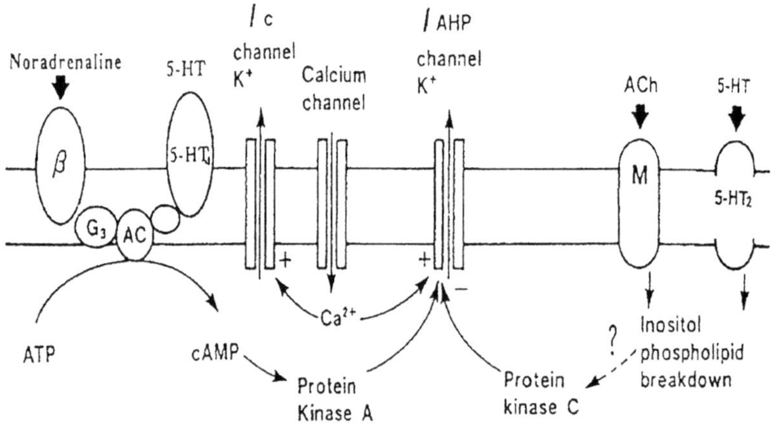

FIG. 7. Schematic representation of Ca^{2+}-activated K^+ channel and intracellular signal transduction systems involved in the monoaminergic modulation of the excitability of postsynaptic neurons. *AC*, adenylate cyclase; *ACh*, acetylcholine; *AHP*, afterhyperpolarization; *β*, β-adrenergic receptor; *M*, muscarinic receptor

comparison with the effects when the same drugs were added acutely to the bathing medium.

These results suggest that chronic treatment with monoamine reuptake inhibitors may enhance the activity of PKA, which inhibits the slow AHP via phosphorylation of Ca^{2+}-activated K^{+} channels. Inhibition of the slow AHP in the cortical neurons might be a common physiological function of the central noradrenergic and serotonergic nervous system. McCormick and colleagues (1991), using hippocampal slice preparations from human temporal lobe tissue suggested that the enhancement of neuronal excitability via the inhibition of the slow AHP might be a common physiological function in the central noradrenergic and serotonergic nervous systems (Fig. 8).

These electrophysiological studies demonstrated enhancement of monoaminergic neurotransmission after chronic antidepressant treatment, despite the down-regulation of postsynaptic receptors. On the other hand, we have shown the suppression of stress-induced increase in monoamine metabolism by antidepressants in the forced-swimming test combined with in vivo brain microdialysis. Subacute treatment with tricyclic antidepressants, SSRIs, and electroconvulsive shock significantly shortened the duration of immobility elicited by forced swimming. In parallel with the behavioral changes, these treatments also significantly suppressed the increase in dopamine and 5-HT in the hypothalamus induced by forced swimming. These results suggest that the pharmacologically different antidepressant drugs may exert their clinical efficacy through the gradual increase in synaptic availability of monoamine without any activation of monoaminergic firings and the net increase in the postsynaptic cascade of signal transduction (Menkes et al. 1983).

Conclusion

Many clinicians strongly hope for the development of novel antidepressants that have more rapid clinical action and effectiveness than the antidepressants now available. To develop such drugs, it is necessary to elucidate which plastic changes in the neurons after chronic antidepressant treatment may be involved in the mechanism of the antidepressant action. Since the discovery of the down-regulation of postsynaptic β-adrenergic receptors, many researchers have supposed that the net decrease in noradrenergic neurotransmission after chronic antidepressant treatment might be involved in their mechanism of action.

However, we suppose that the improvement in synaptic efficacy in serotonergic and/or noradrenergic neurons without excitation of the activity of presynaptic neurons may be a final common pathway of clinically effective antidepressant treatment. Such a net increase in noradrenergic and/or serotonergic neurotransmission may normalize the S/N ratio in the cerebral cortical neurons. Therefore, drugs that rapidly induce the down-regulation of autoreceptors or directly activate intracellular signal-transduction systems

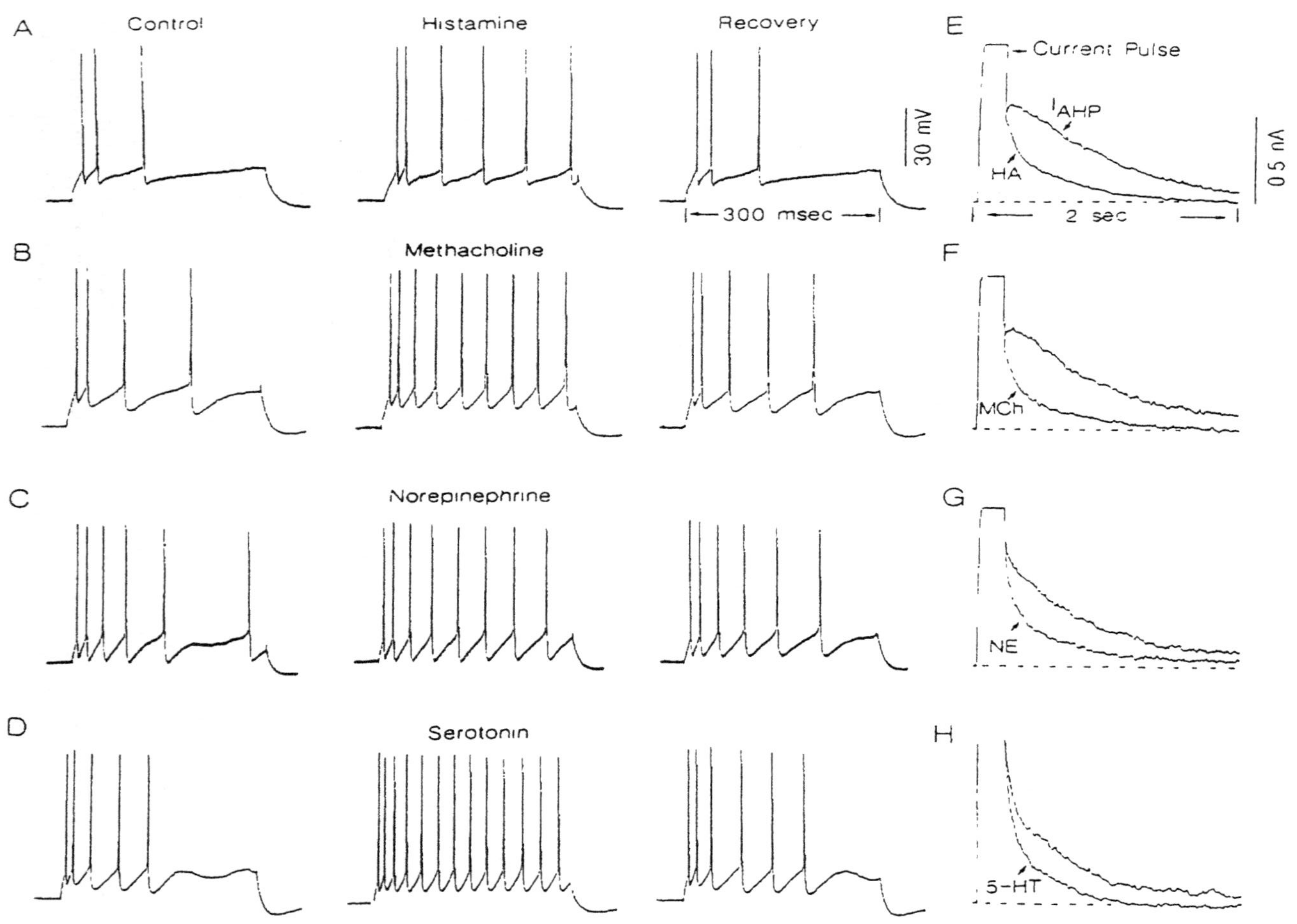

FIG. 8. Effects of histamine (*HA*) methacholine (*MCh*) norepinephrine (*NE*), and serotonin (*5-HT*) on spike frequency adaptation and Ca^{2+}-activated potassium current (I_{AHP}) in human neocortical neurons recorded in vitro (Reprinted from McCormick et al., Neurobiology of the locus coeruleus, 1991, pp 293–305, with kind permission of Elsevier Science – NL, Sara Burgerhartstraat 25, 1055 KV Amsterdam, The Netherlands)

may be rapidly acting and more effective drugs. These drugs may be the most promising novel antidepressants, although their specificity of action and adverse effects are problematic.

References

Andrade R, Nicoll RA (1987) Pharmacologically distinct action of serotonin on single pyramidal neurons of the rat hippocampus recorded in vitro. J Physiol 394:99–124

Birnbaumer L (1990) G proteins in signal transduction. Annu Rev Pharmacol Toxicol 30:675–705

Blakely RD, Berson HE, Fremau RT Jr, Caron MG, Peek MM, Prince HK, Bradley CC (1991) Cloning and expression of a functional serotonin transporter from rat brain. Nature 354:66–70

Blier P, De Montigny C, Chaput Y (1990) A role for the serotonin system in the mechanisms of action of antidepressant treatments: preclinical evidence. J Clin Psychiatry 51S:14–20

Brunello N, Langer SZ, Perez J, Racagni G (1994/1995) Current understanding of the mechanism of action of classic and newer antidepressant drugs. Depression 2:119–126

Chaput Y, De Montigny C, Blier P (1991) Pre- and postsynaptic modifications of the serotonin system by long-term administration of antidepressant treatments: an in vivo electrophysiological study in the rat. Neuropsychopharmacology 5:219–229

Cohen JD, Servan-Schreiber D (1993) A theory of dopamine function and its role in cognitive deficits in schizophrenia. Schizophr Bull 19:85–104

De Montigny C, Aghajanian GK (1978) Tricyclic antidepressants: long term treatment increases responsiveness of rat forebrain neurons to serotonin. Science 202:1303–1306

De Montigny C, Chaput Y, Blier P (1990) Modification of serotonergic neuron properties by long-term treatment with serotonin reuptake blockers. J Clin Psychiatry 51 (Suppl B):4–8

Gilman AG (1987) G proteins: transducers of receptor-generated signals. Annu Rev Biochem 56:615–649

Hoffman BJ, Mesey E, Brownstein M (1991) Cloning of a serotonin transporter affected by antidepressants. Science 254:579–580

Kasper S, Lepine JP, Mendlewicz J, Montgomery SA, Rush AJ (1994/1995) Efficacy, safety, and indications for tricyclic and newer antidepressants. Depression 2:127–137

Köhler M, Hirschberg B, Bond TC, Kinzie JM, Marrion NV, Maylie J, Adelman JP (1996) Small-conductance, calcium-activated potassium channels from mammalian brain. Science 273:1709–1714

Lecrubier Y (1993) Antidepressant drugs: similar but different? In: Mendlewicz J, Brunello N, Langer SZ, Racagni G (eds) New pharmacological approaches to the therapy of depressive disorders. Karger, Basel (International Academy for Biomedical and Drug Research), vol 5, pp 83–910

Madison DV, Nicoll RA (1982) Noradrenaline blocks accommodation of pyramidal cell discharge in the hippocampus. Nature 299:636–638

McCormick DA, Pape H, Williamson A (1991) Action of norepinephrine in the cerebral cortex and thalamus: Implications for function of the central noradrenergic system. In: Barnes CD, Pompeiano O (eds) Neurobiology of the locus coeruleus. (Progress in brain research, vol 88) Elsevier, Amsterdam, pp 293–305

Menkes DB, Rasenick MM, Wheeler MA, Bitensky NW (1983) Guanine triphosphate activation of brain adenylate cyclase: enhancement by long-term antidepressant treatment. Science 129:65–67

Pacholczyk T, Blakely RD, Amara SG (1991) Expression cloning of a cocaine and antidepressant-sensitive human noradrenaline transporter. Nature 350:350–354

Scuvee-Moreau JJ, Dresse AE (1979) Effects of various antidepressant drugs on the spontaneous firing rate of locus coeruleus and dorsal raphe neurons of the rats. Eur J Pharmacol 57:219–225

Sugrue MF (1983) Do antidepressants possess a common mechanism of action? Biochem Pharmacol 12:1811–1817

Sulser F (1984) Antidepressant treatments and regulation of norepinephrine-receptor-coupled adenylate cyclase systems in brain. Adv Biochem Psychopharmacol 39:249–261

Worley PF, Baraban JM, Snyder SH (1987) Beyond receptors: multiple second messenger systems in brain. Neurol Prog 21:217–229

Serotonin-2A Receptor Function in Affective Disorders

Ichiro Kusumi and Tsukasa Koyama

Introduction

Serotonin (5-hydroxytryptamine, 5-HT) has a significant, but certainly not exclusive, role in the core behaviors that are disturbed in affective disorders (e.g., mood, sleep, sexual activity, appetite, circadian and seasonal rhythms, neuroendocrine function, body temperature, motor activity, and cognitive function (Meltzer and Lowy 1987). There has been especially extensive interest in central 5-HT_2 receptor dysfunction as an important factor in the etiology of affective disorders.

The 5-HT_{2A} receptor is one of three subtypes that comprise the 5-HT_2 family of 5-HT receptors according to the nomenclature system introduced by Martin and Humphrey (1994). 5-HT_{2A}, 5-HT_{2B}, and 5-HT_{2C} receptors share more than 60% amino acid sequence homology and couple preferentially to activation of phospholipase C. Herein the original 5-HT_2 receptors are referred to as 5-HT_{2A} receptors; the 5-HT_{1C} receptors are referred to as 5-HT_{2C} receptors.

Role of 5-HT_{2A} Receptor Function in Etiology of Affective Disorders

Postmortem Brain Studies

Several investigators have indicated increased 5-HT_{2A} receptor density in the frontal cortex of depressed patients (McKeith et al. 1987; Yates et al. 1990) and suicide victims (Mann et al. 1986; Arora and Meltzer 1989a), as shown in Table 1. However, these findings have not always been confirmed (Owen et al. 1986; Cheetham et al. 1988). Differences among the studies may be due to

Department of Psychiatry, Hokkaido University School of Medicine, North 15, West 7, Kita-ku, Sapporo, Hokkaido 060, Japan

TABLE 1. 5-HT_{2A} receptor binding in postmortem brain

Study	Ligand	Subject	Site	Result
McKeith et al. (1987)	[^{3}H]Ket	Major depressive disorder	FC	↑
Cheetham et al. (1988)	[^{3}H]Ket	Depressed suicide victims	FC, TC, OC	→
Yates et al. (1990)	[^{3}H]Ket	Major depressive disorder	FC	↑
Mann et al. (1986)	[^{3}H]Spip	Suicide victims	FC	↑
Owen et al. (1986)	[^{3}H]Ket	Suicide victims	FC, OC	→
Arora & Meltzer(1989a)	[^{3}H]Spip	Suicide victims	FC	↑

Ket, ketanserin; Spip, spiperone; FC, frontal cortex; TC, temporal cortex; OC, occipital cortex.

drug effect (treatment with antidepressants and antipsychotic agents, reducing the 5-HT_{2A} binding), use of different ligands, the postmortem interval, or the heterogeneity of psychiatric illnesses and personality disorders associated with suicide.

Neuroendocrine Studies

Because the secretion of hormones such as cortisol and prolactin can be influenced by 5-HT, one strategy for assessing central serotonergic function in vivo is to measure these hormones following administration of 5-HT precursors and direct or indirect 5-HT agonists. There is strong evidence to suggest that 5-HT_{1A} and 5-$HT_{2A/2C}$ receptors stimulate cortisol and prolactin in humans (Maes and Meltzer 1995).

Several investigators have reported blunted prolactin responses to intravenous L-tryptophan (L-TRP) during depression (Koyama and Meltzer 1986; Deakin et al. 1990). The blunted prolactin responses to L-TRP may reflect abnormalities in the synthesis of 5-HT from L-TRP, its release or reuptake, or decreased responsivity of 5-HT receptors that may mediate the serotonergic influence on prolactin secretion (e.g., 5-HT_{1A} post-synaptic receptors). Subjects with major depression show blunted cortisol or adrenocorticotropic hormone (ACTH) responses following 5-HT_{1A} agonist ipsapirone challenge compared to normal controls (Maes and Meltzer 1995). These results indicate that 5-HT_{1A} postsynaptic receptors are probably down-regulated during major depression.

On the other hand, the cortisol response to oral D,L-5-hydroxytryptophan has been reported to be enhanced in nonmedicated depressed and manic patients (Meltzer et al. 1984). This enhanced cortisol response may be due to increased sensitivity of 5-$HT_{2A/2C}$ receptors, which would be unaffected by 5-HT_{1A} receptor subsensitivity (Maes and Meltzer 1995). Because there is no specific evidence as yet for 5-HT_{2C} receptor supersensitivity during depression, it is suggested that the above results are compatible with up-regulation or supersensitivity of 5-HT_{2A} receptors.

TABLE 2. 5-HT_{2A} receptor binding in platelets

Study	Ligand	Subject	Result	
			Nonmedicated	Treated
Biegon et al. (1987)	[^{3}H]Ket	Depressed	↑	→
Cowen et al. (1987)	[^{125}I]LSD	Depressed	→	↑
Arora and Meltzer (1989b)	[^{3}H]LSD	Depressed	↑	
Pandey et al. (1990)	[^{125}I]LSD	Depressed (suicide attempt)	↑	
Biegon et al. (1990)	[^{3}H]Ket	Suicidal	↑	

LSD, lysergic acid diethylamide.

Platelet Studies

The human platelet has been suggested as a possible model for the central serotonergic neuron because the characteristics of 5-HT uptake, imipramine binding site, 5-HT_{2A} receptor and its second messenger system are similar in platelets and the central nervous system (CNS) (Pletscher 1988). It is not easy to study 5-HT_{2A} receptor function directly and longitudinally in the CNS of depressed patients; therefore platelet 5-HT_{2A} receptors have been used as a peripheral model for brain 5-HT_{2A} receptors. It had not been clear whether the platelet 5-HT_{2A} receptor is identical to the brain 5-HT_{2A} receptor until Cook et al. (1994) reported that the primary structure of human platelet 5-HT_{2A} cDNA is identical to that reported for the human frontal cortex 5-HT_{2A} receptor.

Table 2 summarizes the various findings on 5-HT_{2A} receptor density in platelets from depressed patients with or without a suicide attempt. Three studies indicated increased 5-HT_{2A} receptor density in the platelets of depressed patients compared with those of normal controls (Biegon et al. 1987; Arora and Meltzer 1989b; Pandey et al. 1990); one study did not confirm these findings (Cowen et al. 1987). It has also been reported that 5-HT_{2A} receptor functions were increased in the platelets of nonmedicated depressive patients as measured by 5-HT-stimulated phosphoinositide hydrolysis (Mikuni et al. 1991) and 5-HT-induced aggregation (Brusov et al. 1989).

Calcium Mobilization and Affective Disorders

Phospholipase C (PLC), a membrane-bound enzme, catalyzes degradation of the inositol lipid phosphatidylinositol 4,5-bisphosphate (PIP_2), with the production of inositol 1,4,5-triphosphate (IP_3) and diacylglycerol (DAG) (Fig. 1). IP_3 mobilizes Ca^{2+} from an intracellular storage site by interacting with specific receptors. Ca^{2+} induces multiple responses in the cell, including activation of

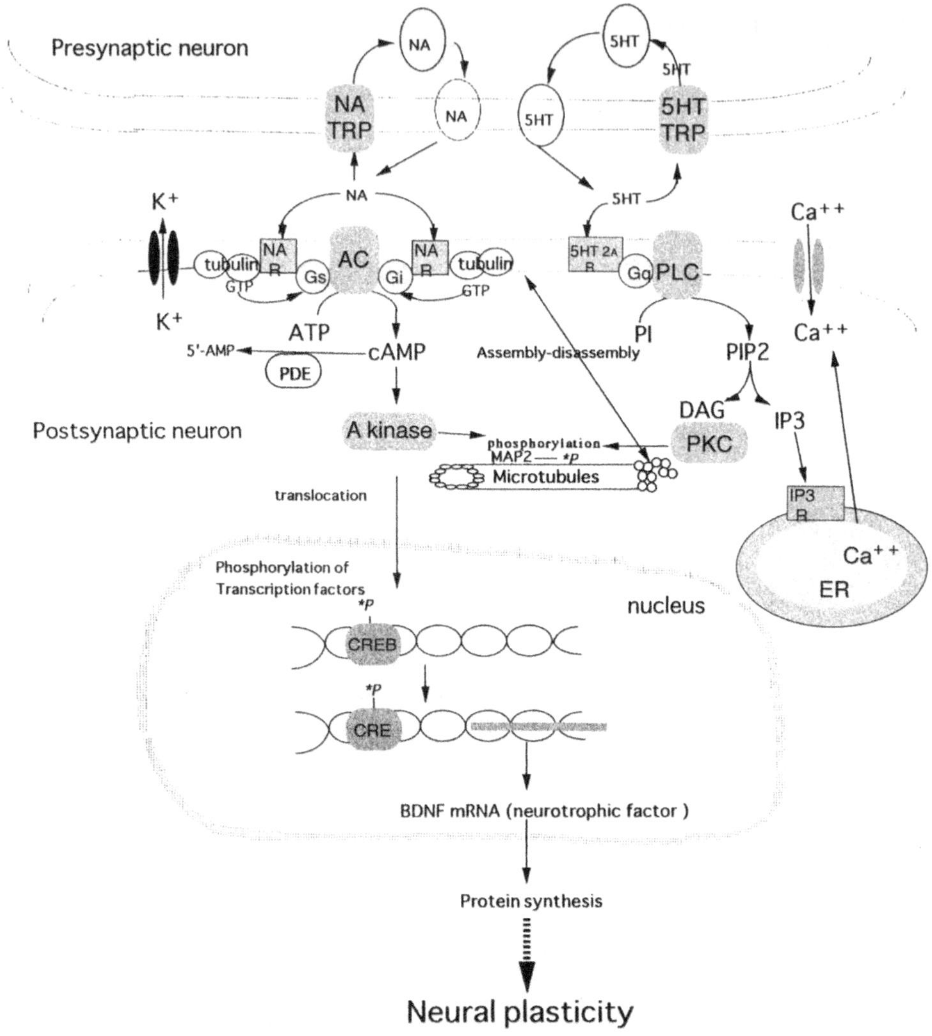

FIG. 1. Signal transduction in the brain. *AC*, adenylate cyclase; *DAG*, diacylglycerol; *ER*; endoplasmic reticulum; *5HT*; serotonin; *IP3*, inositol 1,4,5-triphosphate; *NA*, noradrenalin; *PI*, phosphoinositide; *PIP2*, phosphatidylinositol 4,5-bisphosphate; *PKC*, protein kinase C; *PLC*, phospholipase C; *R*, receptor; *TRP*, transporter

calcium/calmodulin-dependent protein kinases, enzymes that phosphorylate/dephosphorylate key protein substrates in the cell. DAG activates another kinase family, protein kinase C (PKC), which regulates numerous processes of cell function. DAG is also hydrolyzed by a specific lipase to release arachidonic acid with the subsequent formation of prostaglandins and prostacyclins. Thus PLC activation induces diverse changes in the cell, leading to the regulation of many cellular processes (Sanders-Bush and Canton 1995).

In human platelets, stimulation of 5-HT_{2A} receptors has also been suggested to increase phosphoinositide hydrolysis (De Chaffoy de Courcelles et al. 1985), producing IP_3, which mobilizes intracellular calcium ions from internal storage sites (Affolter et al. 1984). Using the Ca-sensitive fluorescent probe fura-2, 5-HT-induced intracellular Ca mobilization in human platelets has been indicated to be mediated by the 5-HT_{2A} receptor (Kagaya et al. 1990). Moreover, it has been shown that the 5-HT_{2A} receptor-mediated Ca response is not significantly affected by sampling time, sampling season, gender difference, age, meals, or exercise in healthy subjects (Kusumi et al. 1991a). Therefore the 5-HT-stimulated Ca response in human platelets is a stable parameter and appears to be suitable for assessing 5-HT_2 receptor function in depressed patients.

5-HT-Induced Calcium Response in Nonmedicated Depressed Patients

Platelet intracellular Ca mobilization after stimulation with 5-HT was measured in nonmedicated patients to compare subgroups of depressed patients with normal subjects and to examine the relation between the Ca response and the severity of depressive symptoms. Informed consent was obtained from all patients and normal subjects. A group of 60 nonmedicated depressed patients were subtyped as 16 with bipolar disorder, 26 with major depression with melancholia, and 18 with major depression without melancholia, according to criteria in the *Diagnostic and Statistical Manual of mental Disorders, Third Edition, Revised* (*DSM-III-R*). For at least 4 weeks before blood sampling they had not received psychotropic medication or any other drug (e.g., aspirin) that might interfere with platelet aggregation. They were all free of physical illness, including hypertension. The severity of their depressive symptoms was assessed by the 21-item Hamilton Rating Scale for Depression (HRSD) at the time of sampling. The clinical data for subgroups of nonmedicated patients are shown in Table 3. Thirty normal control volunteers were hospital or laboratory staff with an age and sex distribution similar to that of the experimental groups. They were all drug-free and had no history of physical or psychiatric illness. Platelet isolation and the measurement of intracellular Ca^{2+} concentration were performed as described previously (Kusumi et al. 1991a, 1991b).

The maximal Ca response induced by 10 μM 5-HT was significantly greater in nonmedicated patients with bipolar disorder and melancholic major depression than in those with nonmelancholic major depression and normal controls (Table 3). The Ca mobilization stimulated by a lower concentration [0.3 μM, approximately 50% effective concentration (EC_{50})] of 5-HT was also significantly higher in the former two groups than in normal controls (Table 3). On the other hand, there were no significant differences among the three subgroups and controls for basal intracellular Ca^{2+} concentration (Table 3).

TABLE 3. 5-HT-induced Ca response in unmedicated depressive patients and normal controls

Parameter	Bipolar disorder	Major depression		Control
		With melancholia	Without melancholia	
No. of patients	16	26	18	30
Age (years)	39.8 ± 3.3	42.9 ± 3.0	40.7 ± 3.6	42.8 ± 2.0
Onset (years)	29.4 ± 2.7	38.5 ± 3.0	36.7 ± 4.1	
Duration (months)	1.9 ± 0.5	3.5 ± 0.7	6.2 ± 2.3	
Family history	2 (13%)	6 (23%)	5 (28%)	
HRSD	23.9 ± 1.3	25.5 ± 1.1	22.2 ± 1.0	
Basal Ca concentration (nM)	71.5 ± 4.4	67.6 ± 2.5	68.3 ± 3.5	76.2 ± 2.4
Ca increase (nM)				
0.3 μM 5-HT	55.2 ± 4.7*	54.9 ± 3.6*	32.7 ± 3.2*	44.2 ± 2.4
10.0 μM 5-HT	122.9 ± 8.7**	113.7 ± 5.8*	77.9 ± 7.2	93.8 ± 3.9

Ca, calcium; HRSD, Hamilton Rating Scale for Depression; 5-HT, 5-hydroxytryptamine (serotonin).
* $P < 0.05$ vs control; ** $P < 0.01$ vs control.

One of our interests was to determine if the magnitude of the Ca response to 5-HT was related to the severity of the depressive symptoms. No relation to the overall psychopathologic process was present, as indicated by the lack of significant correlation between the 5-HT-induced Ca response and the total HRSD score in nonmedicated patients ($n = 60, r = 0.18, p = 0.17$). There were also no significant correlations between the Ca response and each HRSD item in the depressed patients (data not presented).

Change in 5-HT-Induced Calcium Response During Drug Treatment

Repeating the measurement over an extended period in the same nontreated patients might help clarify whether the findings reported here represent state- or trait-dependent variables, but there are practical and ethical difficulties with this approach. Another approach would be to examine the effect of treatment on the Ca response in the same patients. There were seven patients in whom we could measure repeatedly the 5-HT (10 μM)-stimulated Ca mobilization before and during drug treatment. The changes in Ca response and clinical state during the course of the treatment are indicated in Table 4. In cases 2 and 4 the elevated Ca response to 5-HT normalized after remission, but in five of the seven patients the increased Ca mobilization did not change following successful treatment with a variety of drugs that failed to affect this response in vitro and ex vivo (Kusumi et al. 1991a, 1994b).

There were too few subjects to determine a correlation between clinical response and 5-HT-stimulated Ca mobilization, so we next examined the Ca response in euthymic patients whose diagnosis had been previously confirmed

TABLE 4. Change in 5-HT-induced Ca response during drug treatment

Case	Sex	Age (years)	Diagnosis	Increase in Ca response (nM)		
				1st Assay	2nd Assay	3rd Assay
1	F	59	Bipolar disorder	136.7 (27) free	181.1 (HM) Li + HPD	140.2 (Eu) Li
2	M	21	Bipolar disorder	104.4 (24)free	93.3 (0) map	
3	F	41	Major depression with melancholia	130.0 (30) free	134.9 (5) CMI	
4	M	61	Major depression with melancholia	158.0 (35) free	126.1 (21) CMI	70.9 (0) map
5	F	67	Bipolar disorder	149.8 (HM) free	129.6 (Eu) CBZ	
6	M	57	Major depression with melancholia	104.3 (24) fluv	103.5 (2) map	
7	F	66	Major depression with melancholia	179.4 (15) map	170.7 (0) map	

Numbers in parentheses represent the HRSD score.
HM, hypomanic; Eu, euthymic; free, drug-free; Li, lithium carbonate; HPD, haloperidol; map, maprotiline; CMI, clomipramine; CBZ, carbamazepine; fluv, fluvoxamine.

as bipolar disorder ($n = 9$) or melancholic major depression ($n = 8$) and whose HRSD score was less than 5 at the time of sampling. They were treated with the drugs that failed to affect the 5-HT-induced Ca response in vitro and ex vivo in human platelets. The 5-HT (10 μM)-stimulated Ca increase in euthymic bipolar patients was not significantly different from that in nonmedicated patients (Table 5). A similar result was observed for patients with melancholic major depression (Table 5).

Other Calcium Studies

Table 6 summarizes the various findings on resting Ca^{2+} concentration and agonist-stimulated Ca mobilization in the platelets of patients with affective disorders. Most investigators have reported that 5-HT-induced Ca mobilization is increased in platelets from depressed or manic patients (Kusumi et al. 1991b, 1994a; Mikuni et al. 1992; Eckert et al. 1993; Okamoto et al. 1994), although one study did not confirm these findings (Bothwell et al. 1994). The resting intraplatelet Ca^{2+} concentration in bipolar depressed patients is controversial. Dubovsky et al. (1989, 1991) reported that the baseline intracellular Ca level was significantly higher in nontreated depressed bipolar patients than in normal controls. This result fails to agree with our report that there is no significant difference between the two groups (Kusumi et al. 1991b, 1992, 1994a). Tan et al. (1990) indicated that the basal Ca concentration was higher in lithium-treated euthymic bipolar patients than in controls. The lack of

TABLE 5. 5-HT-stimulated Ca response in nonmedicated and euthymic patients with bipolar disorder and melancholic major depression

Parameter	Nonmedicated	Euthymic
Bipolar disorder		
Basal concentration (nM)	71.5 ± 4.4	74.0 ± 3.5
Increase (nM)		
0.3 μM 5-HT	53.4 ± 4.7	55.6 ± 4.8
10.0 μM 5-HT	120.7 ± 8.4	113.0 ± 10.0
Melancholic major depression		
Basal concentration (nM)	67.6 ± 2.5	65.1 ± 3.1
Increase (nM)		
0.3 μM 5-HT	53.2 ± 3.5	54.9 ± 5.7
10.0 μM 5-HT	110.0 ± 5.9	124.1 ± 15.8

TABLE 6. Intraplatelet calcium mobilization in patients with affective disorders

	Nonmedicated	Treated	Reference
Basal Ca level	BD ↑, UD →	BD →, UD →	Dubovsky et al. (1989, 1991)
		BD ↑	Tan et al. (1990)
	BD →, UD →	BD →, UD →	Kusumi et al. (1991b, 1992, 1994a)
	UD →		Mikuni et al. (1992)
		UD →	Eckert et al. (1993)
	BM →	BM →	Okamoto et al. (1994)
	BUD →	BUD →	Bothwell et al. (1994)
5-HT-induced Ca	BD ↑, UMD ↑, UND →	BD ↑, UMD ↑	Kusumi et al. (1991b, 1994a)
response	UD ↑		Mikuni et al. (1992)
		UD ↑	Eckert et al. (1993)
	BM ↑	BM →	Okamoto et al. (1994)
	BUD →	BUD ↑ →	Bothwell et al. (1994)
Thrombin-induced Ca response	BD ↑, UD →	BD →, UD →	Dubovsky et al. (1989, 1991)
		BD ↑	Tan et al. (1990)
	BD ↑, UMD →, UND →		Kusumi et al. (1992)
	BUD →	BUD →	Bothwell et al. (1994)
NE-induced Ca response	UD →		Mikuni et al. (1992)

NE, norepinephrine; BD, bipolar depression; BM, bipolar mania; BUD, bipolar and unipolar depression; UD, unipolar depression; UMD, unipolar melancholic depression; UND, unipolar nonmelancholic depression.

baseline measurements from the bipolar patients (before treatment) does not allow a conclusive answer to this question. As for the resting Ca level in unipolar depression, no report has shown that there is a significant difference among nonmedicated and treated patient groups and the normal controls (Table 6).

There have been several reports of an intracellular Ca response after stimulation by other agonists (Table 6). Thrombin-induced Ca mobilization is increased in the platelets of nonmedicated bipolar depressed patients compared with that in unipolar depressed patients and normal controls (Dubovsky et al. 1991; Kusumi et al. 1992). Similar results have been obtained in other cells, such as neutrophils stimulated with chemotactic tripeptide formylmethionylleucylalanine (van Calker et al. 1993). These findings suggest the possibility that the PLC-linked second messenger system might generally have an increased sensitivity to agonist stimulation in bipolar depressed patients. On the other hand, there is no significant difference in norepinephrine-stimulated Ca mobilization between nonmedicated unipolar depressed subjects and normal controls (Mikuni et al. 1992). The fact that α_2-adrenergic receptor-mediated Ca response is much less than that induced by 5-HT_{2A} receptor suggests that most of the α_2-adrenergic receptors are associated with the inhibition of adenylate cyclase.

As mentioned above, increased Ca mobilization after 5-HT_{2A} receptor stimulation is not changed following successful treatment of bipolar disorder and major depression with melancholia (Kusumi et al. 1994a). Therefore the enhanced Ca response to 5-HT appears to be trait-dependent rather than state-dependent, as judged by the persistently high level of this parameter after remission and by the lack of significant correlation between the severity of depressive symptoms and the Ca mobilization. Eckert et al. (1993) reported that the 5-HT-induced Ca increase is elevated in depressed patients under antidepressant treatment, which supports our finding. On the other hand, thrombin-stimulated Ca mobilization in euthymic-treated bipolar patients is not significantly different from that in normal controls, suggesting a possible state-dependent change in bipolar depression (Dubovsky et al. 1991). However, it is controversial because there is another report that the thrombin-induced Ca response is higher in lithium-treated euthymic bipolar patients than in normal controls (Tan et al. 1990).

Mechanism of 5-HT_{2A} Receptor Hyperfunction

The above-mentioned findings suggest that 5-HT_{2A} receptor function is enhanced in patients with some affective disorders, such as bipolar disorder and major depression with melancholia. The increase in the effectiveness of 5-HT for activating 5-HT_{2A} receptor to produce intracellular Ca mobilization, phosphoinositide (PI) turnover, and aggregation in depressed patients may be associated with the up-regulation of 5-HT_{2A} receptors due to reduced serotonergic transmission. It is still controversial whether the density of 5-HT_{2A} receptor binding is increased in depressed patients as stated under Platelet Studies, above. In addition, it has been demonstrated that depletion of 5-HT levels with *p*-chlorophenylalanine (PCPA) or 5,7-dihydroxytryptamine had no significant effect on the density of 5-HT_{2A} binding (Conn and Sanders-Bush 1986). Moreover, subchronic treatment with high doses of PCPA results in a significant increase in the 5-HT-stimulated PI response in rat hippocampal slices, whereas low doses of PCPA have no significant effect on the 5-HT response compared to that induced by the vehicle (Kusumi et al. 1990, 1991c). There are no significant differences in 5-HT, norepinephrine, or dopamine content between high- and low-dosage PCPA-treated rat brains (Kusumi et al. 1991c). These findings fail to fit the hypothesis that reduced presynaptic serotonergic transmission directly results in postsynaptic 5-HT_{2A} receptor hyperfunction.

Another possibility is that the increased 5-HT_{2A} receptor function can be explained by enhanced transduction of stimuli through a post-receptor mechanism, for example, coupling between the receptor and the guanosine triphosphate (GTP) binding protein or regulation of a second- or third-messenger pathway involving protein kinase, phosphoprotein, and phospholipid. As mentioned under Other Calcium Studies, above, thrombin-induced Ca mobilization in patients with nonmedicated bipolar depression is higher than in those with nonmedicated major depression with or without melancholia and normal controls (Dubovsky et al. 1991; Kusumi et al. 1992). It is interesting to note the difference in these Ca responses between bipolar and unipolar depressed patients. With bipolar disorder there might be some alterations in intracellular signal transduction that are common to both the 5-HT- and thrombin-induced Ca mobilizing pathways. This possibility is partly supported by the report that hyperfunction of GTP-binding protein is observed in the leukocytes of bipolar patients (Schreiber et al. 1991; Young et al. 1994).

As mentioned above (Fig. 1), DAG, a product of PI hydrolysis, is known to activate PKC (Nishizuka 1986). It has been demonstrated that PKC activators, such as mezerein and phorbol 12-myristate-13-acetate (PMA), inhibit 5-HT-stimulated inositol monophosphate (IP-1) accumulation in human platelets (Fig. 2). Furthermore, a PKC inhibitor 1-(5-iso-quinolinesulfonyl)-2-methylpiperazine dihydrochloride (H-7) prevents the PKC activator-induced inhibition against 5-HT_{2A} receptor-mediated IP-1 accumulation (Fig. 2). Similar results are observed in 5-HT-induced Ca mobilization in human platelets (Kagaya et al. 1990). These results suggest that PKC activation may be involved in the 5-HT_{2A} receptor function mediated by its negative feedback system. Thus it is possible that there may be dysregulation of these feedback systems in bipolar affective disorders.

Alternatively, the enhanced 5-HT_{2A} receptor function might be the result of the hormonal disturbances associated with affective disorders. There is converging evidence from various studies that major depression is characterized by a moderately increased spontaneous hypothalamic-pituitary-adrenal

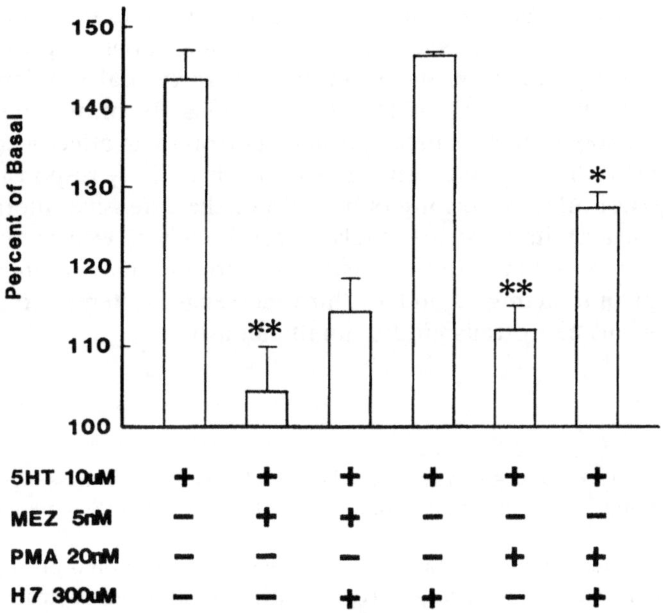

FIG. 2. Effect of H-7 on protein kinase C (PKC) activator-induced inhibition against serotonin (*5-HT*)-stimulated inositol monophosphate (IP_1) accumulation in human platelets. Each value shows the increase from the basal level. The data represent at least four experiments. *Vertical bars* represent the SEM. *MEZ*, mezerein; *PMA*, phorbol 12-myristate-13-acetate. * $P < 0.05$ *vs* 5-HT + PMA; ** $P < 0.01$ *vs* 5-HT only. (With permission from Kagaya et al., 1990)

(HPA) axis function and by failure to suppress plasma intact ACTH and cortisol with the 1 mg dexamethasone suppression test (Maes et al. 1991). Moreover, the important relation between serotonergic activity and the HPA axis has been often discussed (Maes and Meltzer 1995). For example, it has been reported that dexamethasone treatment potentiates 5-HT_{2A} receptor-mediated Ca mobilization in C6 glioma cells, which suggests the possibility that glucocorticoid may act on some modifications in postreceptor mechanisms (Muraoka et al. 1993).

Conclusion

We mainly focused on the dysregulation of 5-HT_{2A} receptor functions in the pathophysiology of affective disorders. Further studies are required to investigate whether the development of enhanced 5-HT_{2A} receptor function in the depressed patients is due to a primary abnormality in the postreceptor mechanism or is secondary to reduced presynaptic function, and whether it is genetically determined or due to environmental factors. Various studies also suggest that alterations in presynaptic 5-HT activity, alterations in postsynaptic 5-HT_{2A} and 5-HT_{1A} receptors in the brain, and reciprocal relations between dysfunctions in these systems and the HPA axis may be of special importance among the biological factors predisposing a person to an affective disorder. It seems doubtful that any one neurotransmitter is entirely responsible for the pathogenesis of affective disorders because of the extensive interactions between neurotransmitters at the levels of cell bodies as well as the terminal regions. It is important in future investigations to continue a strategy of examining multiple interacting second- or third-messenger systems and the balance between various neurotransmitters simultaneously.

References

Affolter H, Erne P, Buergisser E, Pletscher A (1984) Ca^{2+} as messenger of 5-HT_2-receptor stimulation in human blood platelets. Naunyn Schmiedebergs Arch Pharmacol 325:337–342

Arora RC, Meltzer HY (1989a) Serotonergic measures in the brains of suicide victims: 5-HT_2 binding sites in the frontal cortex of suicide victims and control subjects. Am J Psychiatry 146:730–736

Arora RC, Meltzer HY (1989b) Increased serotonin2 (5-HT_2) receptor binding as measured by ^{3}H-lysergic acid diethylamide (^{3}H-LSD) in the blood platelets of depressed patients. Life Sci 44:725–734

Biegon A, Weizman A, Karp L, Ram A, Tiano S, Wolff M (1987) Serotonin 5-HT_2 receptor binding on blood platelets: a peripheral marker for depression? Life Sci 41:2485–2492

Biegon A, Grinspoon A, Blumenfeld B, Bleich A, Apter A, Mester R (1990) Increased serotonin 5-HT_2 receptor binding on blood platelets of suicidal men. Psychopharmacology 100:165–167

Bothwell RA, Eccleston D, Marshall E (1994) Platelet intracellular calcium in patients with recurrent affective disorders. Psychopharmacology 114:375–381

Brusov OS, Beliaev BS, Katasonov AB, Zlobina GP, Factor MI, Lideman RR (1989) Does platelet serotonin receptor supersensitivity accompany endogenous depression? Biol Psychiatry 25:375–381

Cheetham SC, Crompton MR, Katona CLE, Horton RW (1988) Brain 5-HT_2 receptor binding sites in depressed suicide victims. Brain Res 443:272–280

Conn PJ, Sanders-Bush E (1986) Regulation of serotonin-stimulated phosphoinositide hydrolysis; relation to the serotonin 5-HT-2 binding site. J Neurosci 6:3669–3675

Cook EH, Fletcher KE, Wainwright M, Marks N, Yan S-Y, Leventhal BL (1994) Primary structure of the human platelet serotonin 5-HT_{2A} receptor: identity with frontal cortex serotonin 5-HT_{2A} receptor. J Neurochem 63:465–469

Cowen PJ, Charig EM, Fraser S, Elliott JM (1987) Platelet 5-HT receptor binding during depressive illness and tricyclic antidepressant treatment. J Affect Disord 13:45–50

Deakin JF, Pennell I, Upadhyaya AJ, Lofthouse R (1990) A neuroendocrine study of 5-HT function in depression: evidence for biological mechanisms of endogenous and psychosocial causation. Psychopharmacology 101:85–92

De Chaffoy de Courcelles D, Leysen JE, De Clerck F, Van Belle H, Janssen PAJ (1985) Evidence that phospholipid turnover is the signal transducing system coupled to serotonin-S2 receptor sites. J Biol Chem 260:7603–7608

Dubovsky SL, Christiano J, Daniell LC, Franks RD, Murphy J, Adler L, Baker N, Harris A (1989) Increased platelet intracellular calcium concentration in patients with bipolar affective disorders. Arch Gen Psychiatry 46:632–638

Dubovsky SL, Lee C, Christiano J, Murphy J (1991) Elevated platelet intracellular calcium concentration in bipolar depression. Biol Psychiatry 29:441–450

Eckert A, Riemann GD, Aldenhoff J, Mueller WE (1993) Elevated intracellular calcium levels after 5-HT_2 receptor stimulation in platelets of depressed patients. Biol Psychiatry 34:565–568

Kagaya A, Mikuni M, Kusumi I, Yamamoto H, Takahashi K (1990) Serotonin-induced acute desensitization of serotonin2 receptors in human platelets via a mechanism involving protein kinase C. J Pharmacol Exp Ther 255:305–311

Koyama T, Meltzer HY (1986) A biochemical and neuroendocrine study of the serotonergic system in depression. In: Hippius H (ed) New results in depression research. Springer, Berlin Heidelberg, pp 169–188

Kusumi I, Mikuni M, Kuroda Y, Takahashi K (1990) Subchronic administration of para-chlorophenylalanine enhances serotonin-stimulated phosphoinositide hydrolysis in rat hippocampal slices. J Neural Transm 80:181–188

Kusumi I, Koyama T, Yamashita I (1991a) Effect of various factors on serotonin-induced Ca^{2+} response in human platelets. Life Sci 48:2405–2412

Kusumi I, Koyama T, Yamashita I (1991b) Serotonin-stimulated Ca^{2+} response is increased in the blood platelets of depressed patients. Biol Psychiatry 30:310–312

Kusumi I, Mikuni M, Takahashi K (1991c) Effect of subchronic antidepressant administration on serotonin-stimulated phosphoinositide hydrolysis in para-chlorophenylalanine-treated rat hippocampal slices. Prog Neuropsychopharmacol Biol Psychiatry 15:393–403

Kusumi I, Koyama T, Yamashita I (1992) Thrombin-induced platelet calcium mobilization is enhanced in bipolar disorder. Biol Psychiatry 32:731–734

Kusumi I, Koyama T, Yamashita I (1994a) Serotonin-induced platelet intracellular calcium mobilization in depressed patients. Psychopharmacology 113:322–327

Kusumi I, Koyama T, Yamashita I (1994b) Effect of mood stabilizing agents on agonist-induced calcium mobilization in human platelets. J Psychiatr Neurosci 19: 222–225

Maes M, Meltzer HY (1995) The serotonin hypothesis of major depression. In: Bloom FE, Kupfer DJ (eds) Psychopharmacology: the fourth generation of progress. Raven, New York, pp 933–944

Maes M, Vandervorst C, Suy E, Minner B, Raus J (1991) A multivariate study on the simultaneous urinary free cortisol, plasma cortisol, adrenocorticotropic hormone and beta-endorphin escape from suppression by dexamethasone in melancholic patients. Acta Psychiatr Scand 83:480–491

Mann JJ, Stanley M, McBride PA, McEwen BS (1986) Increased serotonin2 and beta-adrenergic receptor binding in the frontal cortices of suicide victims. Arch Gen Psychiatry 43:954–959

Martin GR, Humphrey PPA (1994) Receptors for 5-hydroxytryptamine: current perspectives on classification and nomenclature. Neuropharmacology 33:261–273

McKeith IG, Marshall EF, Ferrier IN, Armstrong MM, Kennedy WN, Perry RH, Perry EK, Eccleston D (1987) 5-HT receptor binding in post-mortem brain from patients with affective disorder. J Affect Disord 13:67–74

Meltzer HY, Lowy MT (1987) The serotonin hypothesis of depression. In: Meltzer HY (ed) Psychopharmacology: the third generation of progress. Raven, New York, pp 513–526

Meltzer HY, Umberkoman-Wiita B, Robertson A, Tricou BJ, Lowy M, Perline R (1984) Effect of 5-hydroxytryptophan on serum cortisol levels in major affective disorders; enhanced response in depression and mania. Arch Gen Psychiatry 41:366–374

Mikuni M, Kusumi I, Kagaya A, Kuroda Y, Mori H, Takahashi K (1991) Increased 5-HT-2 receptor function as measured by serotonin-stimulated phosphoinositide hydrolysis in platelets of depressed patients. Prog Neuropsychopharmacol Biol Psychiatry 15:49–61

Mikuni M, Kagaya A, Takahashi K, Meltzer HY (1992) Serotonin but not norepinephrine-induced calcium mobilization of platelets is enhanced in affective disorders. Psychopharmacology 106:311–314

Muraoka S, Mikuni M, Kagaya A, Saitoh K, Takahashi K (1993) Dexamethasone potentiates serotonin-2 receptor-mediated intracellular Ca^{2+} mobilization in C6 glioma cells. Neuroendocrinology 57:322–329

Nishizuka Y (1986) Studies and perspectives of protein kinase C. Science 233:305–312

Okamoto Y, Kagaya A, Shinno H, Motohashi N, Yamawaki S (1994) Serotonin-induced platelet calcium mobilization is enhanced in mania. Life Sci 56:327–332

Owen F, Chambers DR, Cooper SJ, Crow TJ, Johnson JA, Lofthouse R, Poulter M (1986) Serotonergic mechanisms in brains of suicide victims. Brain Res 362:185–188

Pandey GN, Pandey SC, Janicak PG, Marks RC, Davis JM (1990) Platelet serotonin-2 receptor binding sites in depression and suicide. Biol Psychiatry 28:215–222

Pletscher A (1988) Platelets as models: use and limitations. Experientia 44:152–155

Sanders-Bush E, Canton H (1995) Serotonin receptors: signal transduction pathways. In: Bloom FE, Kupfer DJ (eds) Psychopharmacology: the fourth generation of progress. Raven, New York, pp 431–441

Schreiber G, Avissar S, Danon A, Belmaker RH (1991) Hyperfunctional G proteins in mononuclear leukocytes of patients with mania. Biol Psychiatry 29:273–280

Tan CH, Javors MA, Seleshi E, Lowrimore PA, Bowden CL (1990) Effects of lithium on platelet ionic intracellular calcium concentration in patients with bipolar (manic-depressive) disorder and healthy controls. Life Sci 46:1175–1180

Van Calker D, Foerstner U, Bohus M, Gebicke-Haerter P, Hecht H, Wark H-J, Berger M (1993) Increased sensitivity to agonist stimulation of the Ca^{2+} response in neutrophils of manic-depressive patients: effect of lithium therapy. Neuropsychobiology 27:180–183

Yates M, Leake A, Candy JM, Fairbrairn AF, McKeith IG, Ferrier IN (1990) 5-HT_2 receptor changes in major depression. Biol Psychiatry 27:489–496

Young LT, Li PP, Kamble A, Siu KP, Warsh JJ (1994) Mononuclear leukocyte levels of G proteins with bipolar disorder or major depressive disorder. Am J Psychiatry 151:594–596

Immunological Aspects of Mood Disorders: Interaction Between Cytokines and Intracellular Calcium Signaling

Ariyuki Kagaya and Shigeto Yamawaki

Introduction

The immune system is one of the most important organs, discriminating "self" from "nonself" and protecting "self" from invasion by pathogens or from abnormal "self". The organs of the peripheral immune system are the thymus, spleen, and lymph nodes. The available cells of the immune system include T cells, B cells, and natural killer (NK) cells. Immune responses are typically divided into two components: cellular immunity and hormonal activity by soluble substances such as cytokines. There is increasing evidence of communication among the immune system, the central nervous system (CNS), and the endocrine system at various levels (Jankovic 1994; Dunn 1995). Numerous studies have been published since the 1970s regarding the association between psychological phenomena and immune function. This area of these investigations is now characterized as "psychoneuroimmunology" (Irwin 1995), although there is not sufficient evidence to support interactions between psychological phenomena and immune function. Here we consider the pathophysiology of mood disorders in regard to immune function and demonstrate the importance of intracellular calcium (Ca^{2+}) signaling as a possible factor that associates immune function with psychological phenomena.

Immunological Dysfunction in Mood Disorders

Studies of immunity in those with depression have been conducted since the late 1970s. Numerous reports have been concerned with the evaluation of the number of cells that contribute to the immune system or in vitro cellular immune function (Table 1). Schleifer and colleagues (1989) found that sup-

Department of Psychiatry and Neurosciences, Hiroshima University School of Medicine, 1-2-3 Kasumi, Minami-ku, Hiroshima 734, Japan

TABLE 1. Cellular immune function in depression

Study	Mitogen	Response
Lymphocyte response to mitogens		
Cappel et al. (1978)	PHA	Low
Kronfol et al. (1983)	PHA, ConA, PWM	Low
Schleifer et al. (1984)	PHA, ConA, PWM	Low
Darko et al. (1989)	PHA	Not different
	ConA	Low
Natural killer (NK) cell activity		
Irwin et al. (1987)		Low
Irwin et al. (1990)		Low
Urch et al. (1988)		Low
Kronfol et al. (1989)		Low
Schleifer et al. (1989)		Not different
Darko et al. (1992)		Low
Evans et al. (1992)		Low

PHA, phytohemagglutinin; PWM, pokeweed mitogen; ConA, concanavalin A.

pression of the lymphocyte response to mitogens is associated with the severity of depression. Several other studies failed to find a significant difference in lymphocyte proliferative responses between depressed patients and controls. As for the measurement of NK activity, many studies reported a reduction of NK activity in depressed patients compared to control subjects except for a report from Schleifer et al. (Table 1). Although the findings have been inconsistent and inconclusive, there appears to be a trend toward alteration of cellular immune function in depressed patients.

Another method for determining immune function is to measure cytokine levels following lymphocyte stimulation. Cytokine production by peripheral mononuclear cells in depressed patients has also been described. Maes et al. (1993) reported that depressed patients showed greater accumulation of interleukin-1β (IL-1β, and soluble IL-2 receptor (sIL-2R) from lymphocytes in response to phytohemagglutinin (PHA) and significant correlations between IL-1β production and cortisol values after the dexamethasone suppression test. This result led to a hypothesis that increased production of IL-1β in major depression contributes to the hyperfunction of the hypothalamus-pituitary-adrenocortical (HPA) axis in that illness (Ur et al. 1992). Another study, however, failed to find the higher production of IL-β in response to lipopolysaccharide (LPS); rather, it showed reduced IL-1β production (Weizman et al. 1994).

Stress and Immunological Function

A number of studies have been reported about the relation between psychological stress and the immune system (Biondi and Pancheri 1995). Acute stress, such as examination and disease notification, can be stressors. Chronic

TABLE 2. Effect of chronic psychological stress on immune parameters

Study	Stressor	Result
Bartrop et al. (1977)	Bereavement	Reduction of PHA and ConA response
Schleifer et al. (1983)	Bereavement	Reduction of PHA, ConA, and PWM response
Irwin et al. (1986)	Partner's disease	Impairment of NK cell activity
Kiecolt-Glaser et al. (1987)	Divorce	Reduction of Thelper cells and NK cells

TABLE 3. Effects of cytokines on the CNS

Cytokine	Function
IL-1	Fever elevation, loss of appetite, slow-wave sleep, activation of HPA axis, production of iNOS
IL-2	Release of ACTH and endorphin from pituitary, slow-wave sleep
IL-6	Release of ACTH from pituitary
TNF	Fever elevation, loss of appetite, slow-wave sleep
IFN-α	Fever elevation, loss of appetite, slow-wave sleep, depression

CNS, central nervous system; IL, interleukin; TNF, tumor necrosis factor; IFN, interferon; HPA, hypothalamus-pituitary-adrenal; iNOS; inducible nitric oxide synthese; ACTH, adrenocorticotropic hormone.

stress, such as bereavement, divorce, and life-threatening illness, is also suggested to be an important stressor. These life stressors are capable of disrupting the emotional and affective state of individuals. Several studies have shown the relation between such stress and change in immunological function (Table 2). Psychological stress can change the mental status, compromising immune function.

Fawzy and colleagues (1993) indicated that psychiatric interventions to reduce affective distress have beneficial effects on survival for cancer patients. In that study, modulation of immune function by psychiatric interventions may lead to increased survival.

Alteration of Immune Function and Mood

Cytokines and other products of the immune system play an important role in the communication with the CNS and have various effects on it (Table 3). It has become obvious that glial cells and neuronal cells in the CNS express cytokines and their receptors. Among the various effects of cytokines, it is evident that cytokines can cause mood alteration, such as depression.

For example, not a few patients with human immunodeficiency virus (HIV) infection suffer from depression (Atkinson et al. 1988; Bornstein et al. 1993). HIV has been shown to induce IL-1 in primary rat brain cultures (Merrill et al. 1992). Such changes in cytokine synthesis may affect neural transmission

TABLE 4. Depressive symptom during IFN treatment

Study	Primary disease	IFN	%
Renault (1987)	Hepatitis	α-2b	5
McDonald (1987)	Hepatitis B, HIV	α-A	63
Kuzel (1990)	T-cell lymphoma	α-2a	33
Meyers (1991)	Cancer	α	57
Thomas (1993)	Neovascularization	α-2a	50
Arthur (1993)	Myeloid leukemia	α-2a	20
Lewis (1993)	Macular degeneration	α-2a	21
Schnittman (1994)	HIV	α-2b (with IL-2)	12
Smith (1994)	Melanoma, renal cancer	α-2a (with IL-2)	76
Kagaya (1997)	Hepatitis C	α, α-2b	19

HIV, human immunodeficiency virus.

TABLE 5. Immune parameters during IFN treatment

Parameter	Control ($n = 5$)	Depressed ($n = 5$)
Hamilton		
Before treatment	3.2 ± 1.8	4.2 ± 0.8
After 6-week treatment	2.2 ± 0.8	10.0 ± 1.0**
Plasma levels		
IFN-α (pg/ml)		
Before treatment	0.0 ± 0.0	59.4 ± 57.5
After 6-week treatment	2.9 ± 2.9	75.8 ± 68.7
sIL-2R (ng/ml)		
Before treatment	1.5 ± 0.2	1.7 ± 0.3
After 6-week treatment	1.8 ± 0.2	1.7 ± 0.4
cGMP (pmol/ml)		
Before treatment	10.1 ± 0.9	22.4 ± 3.6**
After 6-week treatment	8.1 ± 1.1	23.3 ± 4.7*

sIL-2R, soluble IL-2 receptor; cGMP, cyclic guanosine monophosphate.
* $P < 0.05$; ** $P < 0.01$ vs control.

mediated by monoamines or other transmitters and may be responsible for the mood disturbances associated with HIV infection.

The interferons (IFNs) are an important group of cytokines that have antiviral and immunomodulatory effects. They are often used to help recovery from such viral infections as chronic hepatitis B and chronic hepatitis C. Their therapeutic efficacy also has been shown for leukemia, lymphoma, cancer, and Kaposi's sarcoma. However, they also sometimes produce psychiatric side effects, such as insomnia, delirium, depressive mood, and suicide (McDonald et al. 1987; Renault et al. 1987). Table 4 shows the current studies that have described depressive symptoms during IFN therapy.

We have shown that 5 of 26 patients with chronic hepatitis C developed mood disturbance during IFN treatment. We also investigated the relation between depressive symptoms and plasma IFN-α-like immunoreactivity, cy-

TABLE 6. Possible effect of IFN-α on the CNS

Tested substance	Effect
Human postmortem brain	IFN-α antibody positive protein in microglia IFN-α mRNA by polymerase chain reaction
Cultured cells	Production of IFN-α/β-like substance in cultured glial cells Potentiation of corticotropin-releasing hormone production by IFN-α in rat hypothalamus primary culture Induction of iNOS in cultured glial cells
Mouse brain tissue	Binding of IFN-α to opioid receptors
Rat brain tissue	Activation of indoleamine-2,3-dioxygenase after chronic treatment with IFN-α Inhibition of peripheral NK cell activity by intracerebroventricular injection of IFN-α IFN-α specific binding

clic guanosine monophosphate (cGMP), and sIL-2R levels during IFN therapy and found that cGMP levels were increased in the patients who suffered from depression (Table 5) (Kagaya et al. 1997). These results suggest that IFN induces a depressive mood, and that cGMP may be a marker for depression or may reflect anxiety. Although the precise mechanism by which IFN-α causes mood disturbance is not fully understood, several studies suggest an effect on the CNS, such as inducible nitric oxide synthase (iNOS) induction (Table 6).

Cytokines and Nitric Oxide Pathway

The biological functions of nitric oxide (NO) were first demonstrated by Furchgott and Zawadzki (1980) using the cardiovascular system. Because NO is unstable, our knowledge of the function of NO was gained from the characterization of NO synthase (NOS). NOS produces NO from L-arginine, resulting in activation of soluble guanylyl cyclase (sGC). sGC accumulates intracellular cGMP, which can regulate Ca^{2+} channels. Several effects of NO are summarized in Table 7.

Nitric oxide synthase is divided into three subtypes: brain NOS (bNOS), endothelial NOS (eNOS), and iNOS (Bredt 1995). bNOS and eNOS are constitutively expressed and are regulated by intracellular Ca^{2+}, whereas iNOS is independent of intracellular Ca^{2+}. It is well known that lipopolysaccharides (LPS) and cytokines can express iNOS in glial cells and macrophages.

In rodent microglia, treatment with LPS or IFN-γ can produce nitrite. Tumor necrosis factor α (TNF-α) is an enhancer of nitrite generation. IL-1β and IL-6 are also known to produce or enhance NO. In astrocytes after treatment with LPS, intracellular cGMP generation is increased, and the generation is blocked by NOS inhibitors. TNF-α, IL-1β, and IFN-γ also induce or facilitate iNOS. C6 cells, a cell line known to demonstrate astrocytic properties, can

TABLE 7. Possible effects of nitric oxide

Activation of soluble guanylyl cyclase
Adenosine diphosphate ribosylation
Inhibition of reduced nicotinamide adenine dinucleatide phosphate (NADPH) oxidase
Inhibition of adenosine triphosphate synthesis
Inhibition of protein synthesis
Inhibition of platelet aggregation and neutrophil adherence
Relaxation of vessels
Regulation of hormone release
In the CNS
Long-term potentiation
Long-term depression
Regulation of neurotransmitter release
Modulation of neuronal cell death

respond to LPS, IL-1β, TNF-α, and IFN-γ, leading to expression of iNOS (Murphy et al., 1995). Evidence suggests that the expression of iNOS in glial cells is mediated by a pathway via tyrosine kinase activation (Feinstein et al. 1994).

Cytokines and Calcium Function

Another line of evidence suggests that dysfunction of intracellular messenger systems, such as phosphoinositide hydrolysis, protein kinases, and Ca^{2+} signaling is important for the pathophysiology of affective disorders (Berridge 1984; Wachtel 1990; Yamawaki et al. 1995, 1996a).

Our laboratory has reported that serotonin (5-hydroxytryptamine, 5-HT)-2A receptor function in platelets (i.e. 5-HT-induced Ca^{2+} mobilization) is enhanced in nonmedicated patients with affective disorders (Yamawaki et al. 1990, 1996b; Okamoto et al. 1995). Several other studies have indicated that 5-HT-induced Ca^{2+} mobilization of platelets is increased in patients with major depression or bipolar depression. Dubovsky et al. (1989) reported that an increase in platelet $[Ca^{2+}]_i$ produced by thrombin and platelet-activating factor is enhanced in bipolar patients (both manic and depressed) but not in unipolar depressed patients. These authors also found that patients with affective disorders have an increased level of resting $[Ca^{2+}]_i$ in platelets and lymphocytes (Dubovsky et al. 1992). These results (Table 8) indicate that with unipolar depression dysfunction is restricted to 5-HT-2A receptor-mediated Ca^{2+} signaling, whereas Ca^{2+} function is primarily dysregulated with bipolar disorders. Furthermore, several studies have demonstrated the effectiveness of Ca^{2+} channel antagonists against affective disorders (Table 9). Together these results suggest that dysfunction of the intracellular Ca^{2+} signaling mechanism may exist in patients with affective disorders.

TABLE 8. Intracellular Ca^{2+} changes in mood disorders

Study	Disorder	Tool	Basal $[Ca^{2+}]_i$	Agonist	$\Delta[Ca^{2+}]_i$
Yamawaki et al. (1990)	Bipolar disorders	Platelets	~	5-HT	↑
Okamoto et al. (1995)	Mania	Platelets	~	5-HT	↑
Yamawaki et al. (1996)	Major depression	Platelets	~	5-HT	↑
	Bipolar disorders	Platelets	~	5-HT	↑
Kusumi et al. (1991)	Depression	Platelets	~	5-HT	↑
Mikuni et al. (1992)	Major depression	Platelets	~	5-HT	↑
				NE	~
Eckert et al. (1993)	Depression	Platelets	~	5-HT	↑
				Thr	~
Konopka (1996)	Depression	Platelets	~	5-HT	↑
Dubovsky et al. (1989)	Unipolar depression	Platelets	↑	Thr, PAF	~
	Bipolar depression	Platelets	↑	Thr, PAF	↑
	Mania	Platelets	↑	Thr, PAF	↑
Tan et al. (1990)	Bipolar disorders	Platelets	↑	Thr	↑
Dubovsky et al. (1992)	Bipolar disorders	Platelets	↑	ND	
		Lymphocytes	↑	ND	
Kusumi et al. (1992)	Bipolar disorders	Platelets	~	Thr	↑
	Major depression	Platelets	~	Thr	~
Berk et al. (1995)	Bipolar disorders	Platelets	~	5-HT	↑
Bothwell et al. (1994)	Bipolar (remission)	Platelets	~	5-HT	~
	Major depression (remission)	Platelets	~	5-HT	~

$\Delta[Ca^{2+}]_i$, increase in $[Ca^{2+}]_i$; Thr, thrombin; PAF, platelet-activating factor; NE, norepinephrine; ND, not determined; ↑, enhanced; ~, not enhanced.

TABLE 9. Effect of Ca^{2+} antagonists on mood disorders

Study	Drug and dosage	Result
Mania		
Dubovsky et al. (1982)	Verapamil (160–480 mg)	Effective (100%)
Giannini et al. (1984)	Verapamil (320 mg)	Effective as lithium
Caillard (1985)	Diltiazem (120–360 mg)	Effective (71%)
Dubovsky et al. (1986)	Verapamil (160–480 mg)	Effective (71%)
Dose et al. (1986)	Verapamil (320–480 mg)	Effective (88%)
Hoschl et al. (1989)	Verapamil (120–480 mg)	Effective as other treatment
Garza-Trevino (1992)	Verapamil (160–320 mg)	Effective as lithium
Depression		
Kramer et al. (1988)	Nifedipine (20 mg)	Not effective
Hoschl et al. (1989)	Verapamil (240–480 mg)	Not effective
Walden et al. (1995)	Nimodipine (180–270 mg)	Effective

These findings pose a question: Is there any relation between the intracellular Ca^{2+} signaling system and cytokines? To answer this question we investigated the effect of cytokines on the intracellular Ca^{2+} signaling system using cultured cells (Kugaya et al. 1995). In C6 rat glioma cells there exist 5-HT-2A receptors whose activation leads to mobilization of intracellular Ca^{2+} (Kagaya et al. 1993, 1995). When the cells were pretreated with IL-1β, the intracellular Ca^{2+} rise in response to 5-HT was attenuated to approximately 70% (Fig. 1). The attenuating effect of IL-1β was exerted in a dose- and time-dependent manner; and the obvious inhibition was observed several hours after pretreatment with IL-1β. LPS also inhibited 5-HT-induced Ca^{2+} mobilization. The inhibitory effects of IL-1β and LPS were significantly prevented by genistein, a selective tyrosine kinase antagonist (Fig. 1). These results indicate that IL-1β and LPS inhibit 5-HT-2A receptor-mediated Ca^{2+} mobilization via a pathway that includes activation of tyrosine kinase. The possible relation between the 5-HT-induced Ca^{2+} rise and the tyrosine kinase pathway in C6 cells has been confirmed by another substance (Kagaya et al. 1996). The precise mechanisms of the interaction between cytokines and monoamine receptor-mediated Ca^{2+} signaling are still unknown, but a cGMP-dependent pathway and a tyrosine kinase pathway are important candidates (Fig. 2). Dysfunction of the interaction may result in the lack of the attenuating effect on the Ca^{2+} signaling system, leading to enhancement of Ca^{2+} movement.

Conclusion

The foregoing suggests that there is substantial evidence for multidirectional communications among mood, the immune system, and the Ca^{2+} signaling system (Fig. 3). The mechanisms to convert molecular to psychological effects remain unclear. Further investigation is necessary to determine the details of

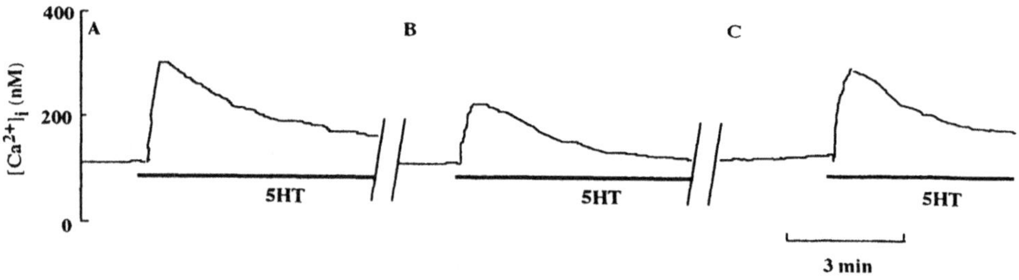

FIG. 1. Effect of interleukin-1β (IL-1β) on serotonin (5-hydroxytryptamine, 5-HT)-induced Ca^{2+} mobilization in C6 cells. The cells were exposed to 10μM 5-HT during the time underlined. (**A**) Cells pretreated with vehicle for 1 day. (**B**) Cells pretreated with IL-1β 10^3 U/ml for 1 day. (**C**) Cells pretreated with IL-1β 10^3 U/ml and 50μM genistein for 1 day

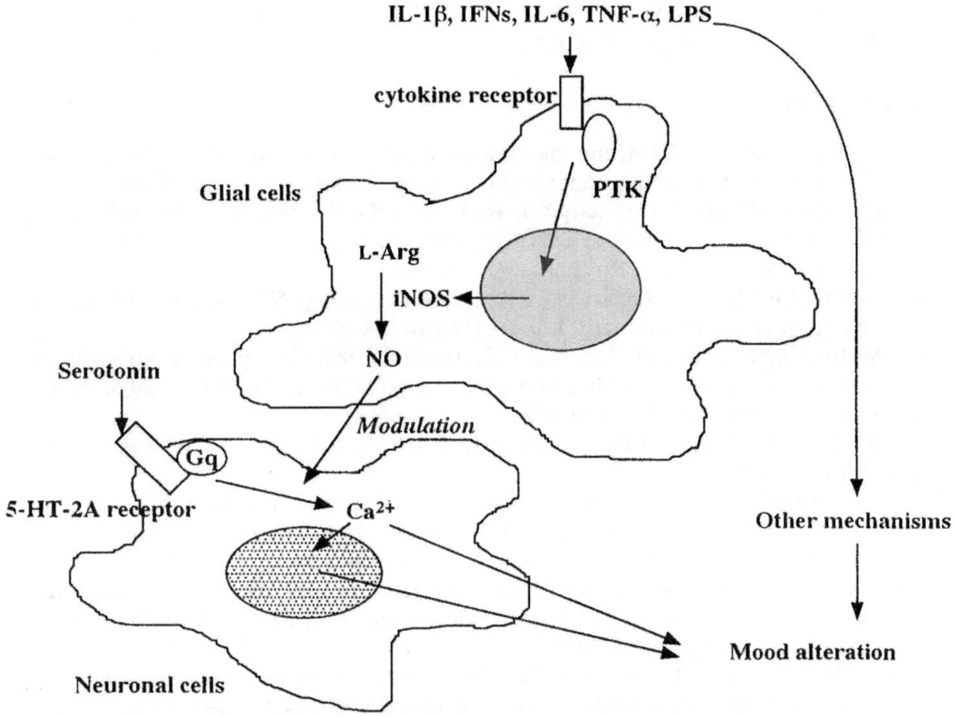

FIG. 2. Possible interaction of cytokine- and neurotransmitter-mediated signaling pathway and mood. *PTK*, tyrosine kinase; *Gq*, GTP-binding protein, Gq type

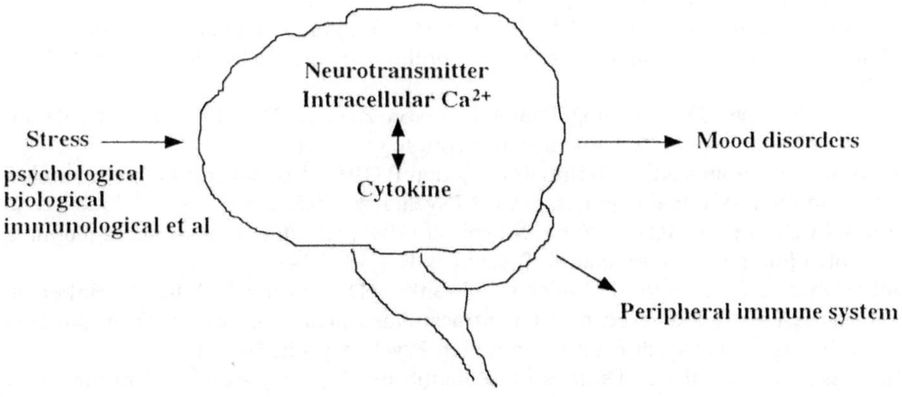

FIG. 3. Hypothesis of psychoneuroimmunology: neurotransmitter–Ca^{2+} signaling and cytokine as mediators of mood regulation

the mechanisms of the communication, as it is important to understand the pathophysiology of mood disorders.

References

Arthur CK, Ma DDF (1993) Combined interferon alfa-2a and cytosine arabinoside as first-line treatment for chronic myeloid leukernia. Acta Haematol 89:15–21

Atkinson JH Jr, Grant I, Kennedy CJ, Richman DD, Spector SA, McCutchan JA (1988) Prevalence of psychiatric disorders among men infected with human immunodeficiency virus. Arch Gen Psychiatry 45:859–864

Bartrop RW, Luckhurst E, Lazarus L, Kikoh LG, Penny R (1977) Depressed lymphocyte function after bereavement. Lancet 1(8016):834–836

Berk M, Bodemer W, van Oudenhove T, Butkow N (1995) The platelet intracellular calcium response to serotonin in augmented in bipolar manic and depressed patients. Human Psychopharmacol 10:189–193

Berridge MJ (1984) Inositol trisphosphate and diacylglycerol as second messengers. Biochem J 220:345–360

Biondi M, Pancheri P (1995) Clinical research strategies in psychoimmunology: A review of 46 human research studies (1972–1992). In: Leonard B, Miller K (eds) Stress, the immune system and psychiatry. Wiley, Chichester, pp 85–111

Bornstein RA, Pace P, Rosenberger P, Nasrallah HA, Para MF, Whitacre CC, Fass RJ (1993) Depression and neuropsychological performance in asymptomatic HIV infection. Am J Psychiatry 150:922–927

Bothwell RA, Eccleston D, Marshall E (1994) Platelet intracellular calcium in patients with recurrent affective disorders. Psychopharmacology 114:375–381

Bredt DS (1995) Molecular characterization of nitric oxide synthase. In: Vincent S (ed) Nitric oxide in the nervous system. Academic, London, pp 1–19

Caillard V (1985) Treatment of mania using a calcium antagonist—preliminary trial. Neuropsychobiology 14:23–26

Cappel R, Gregoire F, Thiry L, Sprecher S (1978) Antibody and cell-mediated immunity to herpes simplex virus in psychotic depression. J Clin Psychiatry 39:266–268

Darko DF, Gillin JC, Risch SC, Bulloch K, Golshan S, Tasevska Z, Hamburger RN (1989) Mitogen-stimulated lymphocyte proliferation and pituitary hormones in major depression. Biol Psychiatry 26:145–155

Darko DF, Irwin MR, Risch SC, Gillin JC (1992) Plasma beta-endorphin and natural killer cell activity in major depression: a preliminary study. Psychiatry Res 43:111–119

Dose M, Emrich HM, Cording-Tommel C, von Zerssen D (1986) Use of calcium antagonists in mania. Psychoneuroendocrinology 11:241–243

Dubovsky SL, Franks RD, Lifschitz ML, Cohen P (1982) Effectiveness of verapamil in the treatment of a manic patient. Am J Psychiatry 139:502–504

Dubovsky SL, Franks RD, Allen S, Murphy J (1986) Calcium antagonists in mania: a double-blind study of verapamil. Psychiatry Res 18:309–320

Dubovsky SL, Christiano J, Daniel LC, Franks RD, Murphy J, Adler L, Baker N, Harris A (1989) Increased platelet intracellular calcium concentration in patients with bipolar affective disorders. Arch Gen Psychiatry 46:632–638

Dubovsky SL, Murphy J, Thomas M, Rademacher J (1992) Abnormal intracellular calcium ion concentration in platelets and lymphocytes of bipolar patients. Am J Psychiatry 149:118–120

Dunn AJ (1995) Interactions between the nervous system and the immune system: Implications for psychopharmacology. In: Bloom FE, Kupfer DJ (eds) Psychopharmacology: the fourth generation of progress. Raven, New York, pp 719–731

Eckert A, Gann H, Riemann D, Aldenhoff J, Muller WE (1993) Elevated intracellular calcium levels after 5-HT2 receptor stimulation in platelets of depressed patients. Biol Psychiatry 34:565–568

Evans DL, Folds JD, Petitto JM, Golden RN, Pedersen CA, Corrigan M, Gilmore JH, Silva SG, Quade D, Ozer H (1992) Circulating natural killer cell phenotypes in men and women with major depression. Relation to cytotoxic activity and severity of depression. Arch Gen Psychiatry 49:388–395

Fawzy FI, Fawzy NW, Hyun CS, Elashoff R, Guthrie D, Fahey JL, Morton DL (1993) Malignant melanoma, effects of an early structured psychiatric intervention, coping, and affective state on recurrence and survival 6 years later. Arch Gen Psychiatry 50:681–689

Feinstein DL, Galea E, Reis DJ (1994) Suppression of glial iNOS expression by tyrosine kinase inhibitors. Ann NY Acad Sci 738: 325–328

Furchgott RF, Zawadzki JV (1980) The obligatory role of endothelial cells in the relaxation of arterial muscle by acetylcholine. Nature 288:373–376

Garza-Trevino E, Overall JE, Hollister LE (1992) Verapamil versus lithium in acute mania. Am J Psychiatry 149:121–122

Giannini AJ, Houser WL Jr, Loiselle RH, Giannini MC, Price WA (1984) Antimanic effects of veraparnil. Am J Psychiatry 141:1602–1603

Hoschl C, Kozeny J (1989) Verapamil in affective disorders: a controlled, double-blind study. Biol Psychiatry 25:128–140

Irwin M, Smith TL, Gillin JC (1987a) Low natural killer cytotoxicity in major depression. Life Sci 41:2127–2133

Irwin M, Daniels M, Smith TL, Bloom E, Weiner H (1987b) Impaired natural killer cell activity during bereavement. Brain Behav Immun 1:98–104

Irwin M, Patterson T, Smith TL, Caldwell C, Brown SA, Gillin JC, Grant I (1990) Reduction of immune function in life stress and depression. Biol Psychiatry 27:22–30

Irwin M (1995) Psychoneuroimmunology of depression. In: Bloom FE, Kupfer DJ (eds) Psychopharmacology: the fourth generation of progress. Raven, New York, pp 983–998

Jankovic BD (1994) Neuroimmunomodulation—from phenomenology to molecular evidence. Ann NY Acad Sci 741:1–38

Kagaya A, Mikuni M, Muraoka S, Saitoh K, Ogawa T, Shinno H, Yamawaki S, Takahashi K (1993) Homologous desensitization of serotonin 5-HT_2 receptor-stimulated intracellular calcium mobilization in C6BU-1 glioma cells via a mechanism involving a calmodulin pathway. J Neurochem 61:1050–1056

Kagaya A, Motohashi N, Kugaya A, Yamaji T, Hayashi T, Okamoto Y, Shinno H, Takebayashi M, Uchitomi Y, Yamawaki S (1995) Cyclic GMP generation mediated by 5-HT-2 receptors via nitric oxide pathway and its effect on the desensitization of 5-HT-2 receptors in C6 glioma cells. J Neural Transm 100:27–38

Kagaya A, Uchitomi Y, Kugaya A, Takebayashi M, Nagaoka I, Muraoka M, Yokota N, Yamawaki S (1996) Differential regulation of intracellular signaling systems by sodium fluoride in rat glioma cells. J Neurochem 66:1483–1488

Kagaya A, Uchitomi Y, Takezaki E, Fukue M, Tsukano K, Kugaya A, Minagawa H, Takebayashi M, Zensho H, Oyamada T, Yamawaki S (1997) Plasma levels of cyclic

GMP, immune parameters and depressive status during interferon therapy: a prospective study in Japan. Neuropsychobiology 35:128–131

Kiecolt-Glaser JK, Fisher LD, Ogrocki P, Stout JC, Speicher CE, Glaser R (1987) Marital quality, marital disruption, and immune function. Psychosom Med 49:13–34

Konopka LM, Cooper R, Crayton JW (1996) Serotonin-induced increases in platelet cytosolic calcium concentration in depressed, schizophrenic, and substance abuse patients. Biol Psychiatry 39:708–713

Kramer MS, Caputo K, DiJohnson L, Mirow A, Sheves P, Sholevar F (1988) Nagative trial of nifedipine in depression. Biol Psychiatry 24:941–960

Kronfol Z, Silva J Jr, Greden J (1983) Impaired lymphocyte function in depressed illness. Life Sci 33:241–247

Kronfol Z, Nair M, Goodson J, Goel K, Haskett R, Schwartz S (1989) Natural killer cell activity in depressive illness: preliminary report. Biol Psychiatry 26:753–756

Kugaya A, Kagaya A, Uchitomi Y, Motohashi N, Yamawaki S (1995) Inhibition of serotonin-induced Ca^{2+} mobilization by interleukin-1β in rat C6BU-1 glioma cells. Brain Res 682:151–156

Kusumi I, Koyama T, Yamashita I (1991) Serotonin-stimulated Ca^{2+} response is increased in the blood platelets of depressed patients. Biol Psychiatry 30:310–312

Kusumi I, Koyama T, Yamashita I (1992) Thrombin-induced platelet calcium mobilization is enhanced in bipolar disorders. Biol Psychiatry 32:731–734

Kuzel TM, Gilyon K, Springer E, Variakojis D, Kaul K, Bunn PA Jr, Evans L, Roenigk HH Jr, Rosen ST (1990) Interferon alfa-2a combined with phototherapy in the treatment of cutaneous T-cell lymphoma. J Natl Cancer Inst 82:203–207

Lewis ML, Davis J, Chuang E (1993) Interferon alfa-2a in the treatment of exudative age-related macular degeneration. Graefe's Arch Clin Exp Ophthalmol 231:615–618

Maes M, Bosmans E, Meltzer HY, Scharpe S, Suy E (1993) Interleukin-1β: a putative mediator of HPA axis hyperactivity in major depression? Am J Psychiatry 150:1189–1193

McDonald EM, Mann AH, Thomas HC (1987) Interferons as mediators of psychiatric morbidity: an investigation in a trial of recombinant α-interferon in hepatitis-B carriers. Lancet 21:1175–1178

Merrill JE, Koyanagi Y, Zack J, Thomas L, Martin F, Chen ISY (1992) Induction of interleukin-1 and tumor necrosis factor alpha in brain cultures by human immunodeficiency virus type 1. J Virol 66:2217–2225

Meyers CA, Scheibel RS, Forman AD (1991) Persistent neurotoxicity of systemically administered interferon-alpha. Neurology 41:672–676

Mikuni M, Kagaya A, Takahashi K, Meltzer HY (1992) Serotonin but not norepinephrine-induced calcium mobilization is enhanced in platelets of affective disorders. Psychopharmacology 106:311–314

Murphy S, Grzybicki DM, Simmons ML (1995) Glial cells as nitric oxide sources and targets. In: Vincent S (ed) Nitric oxide in the nervous system. Academic, London, pp 162–190

Okamoto Y, Kagaya A, Shinno H, Motohashi N, Yamawaki S (1995) Serotonin-induced platelet calcium mobilization is enhanced in mania. Life Sci 56:327–332

Renault PF, Hoofnagle JH, Park Y, Mullen KD, Peters M, Jones DB, Rustgi V, Jones EA (1987) Psychiatric complications of long-term interferon alpha therapy. Arch Intern Med 147:1577–1580

Schleifer SJ, Keller SE, Camerino M, Thornton JC, Stein M (1983) Suppression of lymphocyte stimulation following bereavement. JAMA 250:374–377

Schleifer SJ, Keller SE, Meyerson AT, Raskin MJ, Davis KL, Stein M (1984) Lymphocyte function in major depressive disorder. Arch Gen Psychiatry 41:484–486

Schleifer SJ, Keller SE, Bond RN, Cohen H, Stein M (1989) Major depressive disorder and immunity: role of age, sex, severity, and hospitalization. Arch Gen Psychiatry 46:81–87

Schnittman SM, Vogel S, Baseler M, Lane HC, Davey RT Jr (1994) A phase I study of interferon-α2b in combination with interleukin-2 in patients with human immunodeficiency virus infection. J Infect Dis 169:981–989

Smith MJ, Mouawad R, Vuillemin E, Benhammouda A, Soubrane C, Khayat D (1994) Psychological side effects induced by interleukin-2/α interferon treatment. Psycho-Oncol 3:289–298

Tan CH, Martin AJ, Ermias S, Patricia AL, Charles LB (1990) Effects of lithium on platetet ionic intracellular calcium concentration in patients with bipolar (manic-depressive) disorder and healthy controls. Life Sci 46:1175–1180

Thomas MA, Ibanez HE (1993) Interferon alfa-2a in the treatment of subfoveal choroidal neovascularization. Am J Ophthalmol 115:563–568

Ur E, White PD, Grossman A (1992) Hypothesis: cytokines may be activated to cause depressive illness and chronic fatigue syndrome. Eur Arch Psychiatry Clin Neurosci 241:317–322

Urch A, Muller C, Aschauer H, Resch F, Zielinski CC (1988) Lytic effector cell function in schizophrenia and depression. J Neuroimmunol 18:291–301

Wachtel H (1990) The second-messenger dysbalance hypothesis of affective disorders. Pharmacopsychiatry 23:27–32

Walden J, Frintze J, van Calker D, Berger M, Grunze H (1995) A calcium antagonist for the treatment of depressive episode: single case reports. J Psychiat Res 29:71–76

Weizman R, Laor N, Podliszewski E, Notti I, Djaldetti M, Bessler H (1994) Cytokine production in major depressed patients before and after clomipramine treatment. Biol Psychiatry 35:42–47

Yamawaki S, Sugihara J, Kato T, Hayakawa H, Shimizu M (1990) 5-HT_2 receptor-mediated Ca^{2+} increase in platelets of bipolar disorder. Presented at the 17th Congress of CINP. Abstracts, p 29

Yamawaki S, Kagaya A, Hayakawa H, Okamoto Y, Kugaya A, Takebayashi M, Muraoka M, Uchitomi Y (1995) Pathophysiology of affective disroders: serotonin receptor function and intracellular calcium signaling. In: Takada A, Curzon G (eds) Serotonin in the central nervous system and periphery. Elsevier, Amsterdam, pp 31–39

Yamawaki S, Kagaya A, Okamoto Y, Uchitomi Y, Shimizu M, Nishida A (1996a) Role of intracellular calcium mechanisms in the pathophysiology of affective disorders. In: Shibuya T (ed) International academy for biomedical and drug research, vol 11: Preclinical and clinical strategies for the treatment of neurodegenerative, cerebrovascular and mental disorders. Karger, Basel, pp 106–115

Yamawaki S, Kagaya A, Okamoto Y, Shimizu M, Nishida A, Uchitomi Y (1996b) Enhanced calcium response to serotonin in platelets from patients with affective disorders. J Psychiatr Neurosci 21:321–324

The Role of G Proteins in the Pathophysiology and Treatment of Affective Disorders

Hiroki Ozawa and Naohiko Takahata

Introduction

Guanosine triphosphate (GTP)-binding proteins (G proteins) have been thought of as modulators that multiply signal information from receptors to effectors. G proteins related to membrane signaling have a heterotrimetric structure (α, β, and γ), and the α subunit has a GTP-binding site involved in GTPase activity hydrolyzing GTP to guanosine diphosphate (GDP). Therefore, the G proteins comprise a unique family of protein molecules implicated in the mechanisms switching signal transduction on and off (Simon et al. 1991). Manic-depressive illness is characterized by two phases, the manic and the depressive states, and generally is considered to be in remission in the period between episodes. From its clinical characteristics, it is conceivable that there is some difficulty in emotional adjustment involving the switching mechanisms that accelerate or diminish neurotransmission in the brain. Hence, one might assume that there is a close relationship between G protein as the protein molecule in the on-off signal switching and manic-depressive illness (Fig. 1). Since the amine hypothesis of manic-depressive illness was proposed, various hypotheses concerning the pathophysiology of this disorder have been discussed, along with the complexity of interactions among multiple neural transmission systems, which contrasts with the increase or decrease in single neurotransmitters such as occurs with noradrenaline and serotonin. One of the neurological bases of signal interaction is that different receptors are coupled with the same G protein. Thus the signal information inputs from different receptors interact via G protein (cross-talk). It is also known that receptor sensitivity is diminished when the release of neurotransmitter is prolonged and raised when the release of neurotransmitter is reduced. Thus, G protein has an important role in the regulation of the affinity of receptors for neurotransmitters, stabilizing mood in the face of multiform social stresses.

Department of Neuropsychiatry, School of Medicine, Sapporo Medical University, Chuo-ku, S.1, W.16, Sapporo, Hokkaido 060, Japan

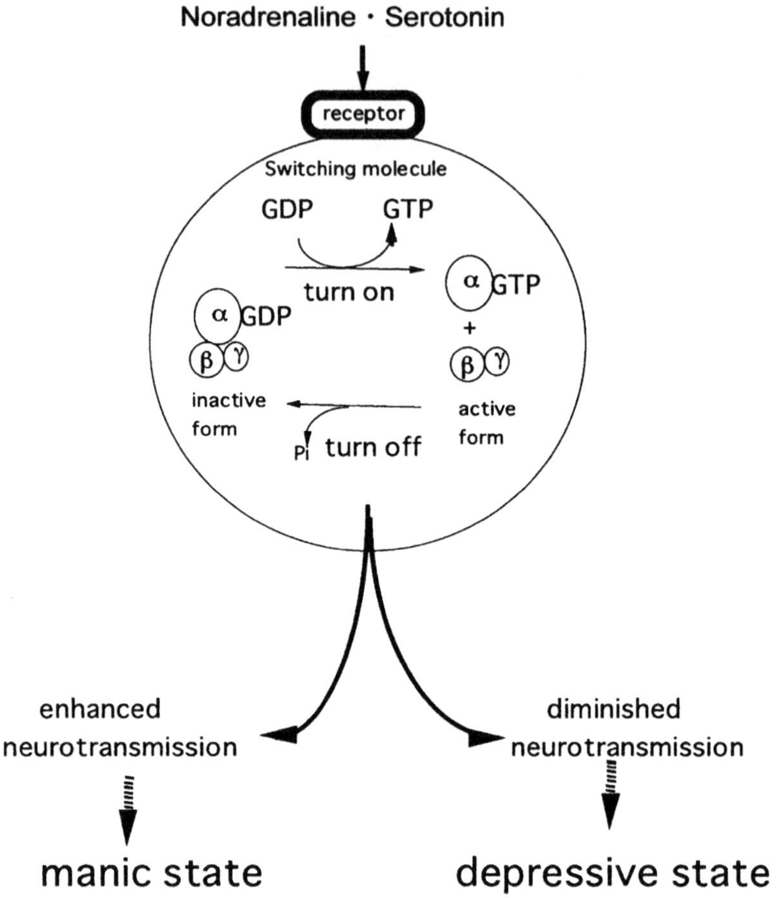

FIG. 1. Monoamine hypothesis and G protein as a switching molecule. *GDP*, guanosine diphosphate; *GTP*, guanosine triphosphate

Changes in the Biological Hypotheses for the Pathophysiology of Manic-Depressive Illness

Table 1 outlines the changing biological hypotheses for the pathophysiology of manic-depressive illness. In the 1960s, it was confirmed that many antidepressants have the ability to inhibit the reuptake of monoamines or monoamine oxidase (MAO). On the basis of this evidence, the monoamine deficiency theory of depression was proposed. However, there are some inconsistencies in this theory:

1. Not all antidepressants have the ability to inhibit the reuptake of monoamine or MAO activity.

TABLE 1. History of research on antidepressant action and hypotheses of depression

Decade	Hypotheses of depression	Mechanisms of antidepressant action
1960s	Monoamine deficiency	Monoamine reuptake inhibition
1970s	Receptor supersensivity	Receptor down-regulation
	Supersensitivity of postreceptor function	Subsensitivity of β-receptor-stimulated cAMP production
1980s	Second-messenger dysregulation	Antidepressant influence on second messenger
1990s	G-protein function imbalance	Antidepressant action on G protein

2. Not all monoamine reuptake inhibitors have antidepressive effects.
3. Experiences with antidepressant therapy have shown that at therapeutic doses, it usually takes 1 to 3 weeks for a clinical response to occur, whereas inhibition of reuptake and inhibition of MAO can appear within minutes after a single dose of active compounds.

In the late 1970s, many researchers focused on postsynaptic adaptation to long-term administration of antidepressants. Down-regulation of β-adrenergic receptors or 5-HT_2 receptors is seen in many cases in which antidepressants are administered for 1 to 2 weeks. In addition, β-adrenergic agonist-induced cyclic AMP production in rat brain slices decreases. These phenomena parallel the lag time for therapeutic benefit seen in the clinical administration of antidepressants. Down-regulation is believed to occur via the homeostatic mechanisms of the neuron, in which prolonged exposure increases monoamine in the synaptic cleft by inhibition of reuptake or inhibition of the antidepressant action by MAO. However, second-generation antidepressants, which do not inhibit monoamine reuptake or catabolism, also induce receptor down-regulation on long-term administration. The receptor supersensitivty hypothesis of depression has been proposed on the basis of this receptor down-regulation. This hypothesis seems to be diametrically opposed to the original monoamine hypotheses. If the receptor supersensitivty hypothesis is true, specific blockers of these receptors might be clinically effective. However, few data support this speculation. Besides, it is reported that selective serotonin inhibitors do not produce receptor down-regulation. Hence, it seems unlikely that a specific neurotransmission system is simply enhanced or diminished by the action of antidepressants. Recently, various neurochemical agents have been shown to act as potent antidepressants. These include selective serotonin uptake inhibitors, γ-aminobutyric acid (GABA)ergic agents, β-adrenergic agonists, phosphodiesterase inhibitors, inositol (a second-messenger precursor), and forskolin analogs (second-messenger activators). Tricyclic antidepressants also act as neurotransmitter receptor-effector systems. These include dopamine, acetylcholine, GABA, and certain peptides.

Furthermore, the mechanisms of action of antidepressants and the pathology of affective disorders involve receptor-G protein-effector function, because G proteins are a key element in the interaction of different neurotransmitters (crossover and cross-talk) and play a critical role in neurotransmission (amplification and deamplication).

Antidepressants and G Proteins

Receptors and G Proteins

Mishra et al. (1980) reported that mianserin caused a significant reduction in noradrenaline-sensitive cAMP production without β-adrenergic receptor down-regulation. This suggests that mianserin induces a change in coupling between β-receptors and G proteins. Okada et al. (1986) reported that desipramine induced uncoupling of Gs from β-receptors before β-receptor down-regulation, indicating that antidepressants may induce uncoupling between β-receptors and Gs. The finding of Hancock et al. (1984) of selective reduction of high-affinity binding sites for β-adrenergic receptors after chronic antidepressant treatment also supported this. However, O'Donnell and Frazer (1985), in isoproterenol displacement experiments, suggested that GTP-induced β-receptor regulation was not changed by chronic antidepressant treatment, unlike β-receptor agonist-induced desensitization. General desensitization phenomena caused by agonist exposure involve a two-step reaction, with functional uncoupling of the receptor and G protein in the early stage and receptor internalization in the late stage. However, no one has confirmed that the mechanism of antidepressant-induced desensitization is the same as that of receptor-agonist stimulation. In contrast to the development and recovery of β-receptor desensitization caused by agonist exposure, antidepressant-induced desensitization is a slow phenomenon. Furthermore, Dibner and Molinoff (1979) reported that β-receptors in brain slices treated with desipramine caused further β-receptor down-regulation during in vitro exposure to an agonist, suggesting that the mechanisms of desensitization phenomena may be different for antidepressant- and receptor-agonist-induced desensitization.

Consequently, the role of β-receptor function in the human brain and the mechanisms of β down-regulation should be reconsidered from the point of view of downstream signal transduction.

G Protein and Adenylyl Cyclase

Menkes et al. (1983) first reported that long-term administration of various antidepressants enhanced guanine nucleotide activation of adenylyl cyclase in rat cortex and hypothalamus membranes. They suggested that this augmentation of adenylyl cyclase was associated with a facilitated G protein-catalytic moiety of adenylyl cyclase. Their idea was apparently inconsistent with the observation that antidepressant-induced subsensitivity of noradrenaline elicited cyclic AMP production in rat brain slices. They explained that this apparent inconsistency was due to the enhancement of α_2-adrenergic inhibition of adenylyl cyclase by interaction between G protein and the catalytic moiety, and that thereby the net accumulation of cyclic AMP was decreased by noradrenaline. There are several reports that GTP analog-, NaF-, or forskolin-stimulated adenylyl cyclase activity is enhanced by long-term antidepressant treatment of membranes. NaF directly stimulates adenylyl cyclase by eliciting the active conformation of Gs protein. The catalytic unit of adenylyl cyclase is a forskolin-binding site with low affinity; however, the high-affinity binding site of that compound reflects the complex of the α subunit of Gs and the catalytic unit of adenylyl cyclase. Hence, forskolin not only stimulates the catalytic unit of adenylyl cyclase but also appears to stabilize the coupling between Gs and the adenylyl cyclase catalytic unit (Seeman 1987). Reports of enhancement of GTP analog-stimulated adenylyl cyclase in membrane preparations followed, but they were inconsistent in that some reported no change in the effects of antidepressants and others reported diminished effects. These contradictory results might be explained by differences in the animal strains used, differences in drugs or in the duration of treatment, or different doses of drugs. However, the adenylyl cyclase assay conditions different more among these studies than did other factors. Interestingly, Newman and Lerer (1989) reported bidirectional results for forskolin-simulated cyclic AMP production of membranes and slice preparations, observing an increase in membranes and a decrease in slices. They suggested that forskolin interacted with different components of the adenylyl cyclase in the two preparations, reflecting the components of the adenylyl cyclase system distal to the receptor affected by chronic antidepressant treatment. Their report is suggestive in the light of the lack of uniformity in results induced by various factors. Slice preparations have tighter coupling of receptors and G proteins than membrane preparations; thus, slice preparations seem to reflect receptor changes or the agonist receptor-G protein coupling state. In contrast, membrane preparations appear to reflect the G protein-effector state distal to the receptor. Even in membrane preparations, there are complicated effects on the receptor-G protein-effector system. Some but not all, investigators report agonist-induced adenylyl cyclase changes in membranes. These differences may be induced by adenylyl cyclase assay conditions involving ATP concentration, ionic concentration, incubation time, or temperature. In some membrane preparations, receptor changes or agonist receptor-G protein coupling states independent of the components distal to the receptor are easy to detect. For example, Duman et al. (1985), Okada et al. (1986), and Tiong and Richardson (1990) were able to detect a decrease in β-agonist-induced cAMP production in a membrane preparation, but not enhancement of G-protein-mediated adenylyl cyclase activity. Our unpublished data suggest that in membrane preparations in which augmentation of guanine nucleotide stimulated by chronic antidepressants is observed, there is no increased effect of β-agonist stimulation on adenylyl cyclase. In our earlier report, we used totally different assay conditions for adenylyl cyclase to determine whether β-agonist promotion of adenylyl cyclase occurred.

Newman and Lerer (1989) also reported that there was no change of isoproterenol-stimulated adenylyl cyclase activity in membrane preparations after chronic antidepressant treatment, but that enhancement of GppNHp-stimulated adenylyl cyclase was observed. The degree of stimulation by isoproterenol was much less in membrane preparations than in slice preparations. Therefore we should select assay conditions for adenylyl cyclase based on whether the effect of the antidepressant is seen proximal or distal to the receptor.

If it is true that G-protein-mediated adenylyl cyclase is enhanced after long-term antidepressant treatment, which postreceptor components are key targets in the action of antidepressants? In general, adenylyl cyclase activity is based on the balance between stimulatory (Gs) and inhibitory (Gi) GTP-binding protein functions. We separately measured the stimulation and inhibition of adenylyl cyclase by GppNHp (Ozawa and Rasenick 1989, 1991). GppNHp-dependent stimulation, but not inhibition of adenylyl cyclase, increased without any change in the affinity of guanine nucleotide for G proteins, suggesting that long-term administration of antidepressants promotes increased coupling between Gs and the catalytic unit of adenylyl cyclase (Ozawa and Rasenick 1989, 1991).

Direct Action on G Protein

One might also expect the change in the amount of G protein to vary in relation to the effect of the antidepressant. Our reports demonstrated that guanine nucleotide binding is unaffected by chronic antidepressant treatment (Ozawa and Rasenick 1989, 1991). Our unpublished data also suggest that adenosine diphosphate (ADP) ribosylation of cholera toxin and pertussis toxin is unchanged. However, one study reported that enzyme-linked immunosaibent assay (ELISA) using various antibodies to G protein α subunits found changes in the amount of G protein caused by chronic antidepressant treatment (Lesch et al. 1991). Our study and other studies did not observe any changes in the quantitation of Gs and Gi α subunits due to chronic treatment with antidepressants, as determined by Western blotting (Cheung and Rasenick 1995; Kamada et al. 1997). These studies did not find changes in the amounts of G proteins. However, it is suggestive that the amounts of G proteins do not parallel the amounts of mRNA; for example, there is 10 times as much Gi and Go than Gs in the brain, but Gs mRNA is abundant. These results indicate that the turnover of Gs protein synthesis is faster than that of Gi and Go. Thus, it does not seem that long-term adaptive action, such as chronic antidepressant treatment, is a reasonable explanation for the synthesis of Gs protein. Additionally, G protein is stable enough for quantitation after developing, even in severe neurodegenerative disease (McLaughlin et al. 1991).

The acute effects of several antidepressants, but not MAO inhibitors, antipsychotics, or anxiolytics, have been demonstrated to increase [^{3}H]GTP binding in a homogenate of rat cerebral cortex. These effects were partially inhibited by pertussis toxin, suggesting that the target sites of antidepressants involve Gi- and Go-like proteins. Furthermore, the same laboratory also reported that the GTPase activity of purified Go and the rate of binding of [^{35}S]GTPγS to the purified protein were increased by antidepressants, indicating that the drugs enhance the dissociation of G protein heterotrimer subunits (Yamamoto et al. 1992). We also examined the in vitro effects of antidepressants on functional photoaffinity labeling of GTP-binding protein. Saturation-binding studies were performed by incubating membranes with increasing concentrations of [^{32}P]AAGTP, followed by UV irradiation and sodium dodecyl sulfate-polyacrylamide gel electrophoresis (SDS-PAGE). The specifically bound isotherms for each of the G proteins studied showed characteristics of a one-site model. Scatchard analysis revealed increases in the B_{max} and K_d of AAGTP binding for each of the G proteins (especially stimulatory G proteins) with the addition of antidepressants such as amitriptyline, clomipramine, desipramine, and mianserin, but not with MAO inhibitors, antipsychotics, or anxiolytics. These results suggested that drugs having antidepressive properties may directly affect G proteins, especially Gs protein (Ozawa et al. 1994).

On the basis of current evidence that cationic amphiphilic compounds, including neuropeptides, antidepressants, and polyamine, directly modify G-protein functions in a receptor-independent fashion, the development of new drugs for the treatment of neuropsychiatric diseases that have G-protein targets is being discussed. Although it will be necessary to extend this preliminary work to a broad spectrum of psychoactive drugs in the near future, we believe the attempt to observe differences in the specificity and selectivity of action sites of psychoactive drugs in each G protein will contribute to the development of novel psychotherapeutics.

Receptor Reconciliation Theory of the Action of Antidepressants

The β- and dopamine-1 receptors appear to be the major Gs-linked receptor types. The observation of down-regulation of these receptors or the supersensitivity of receptor agonist-mediated cyclic AMP accumulation seems to contrast with the observation of guanine-nucleotide-stimulated adenylyl cyclase activity. However, previous work suggests that the receptor coupled to a G protein constrains that G protein (specifically Gs) from interacting with the catalytic subunit of adenylyl cyclase and activating that enzyme. Experiments with permeable C6 glioma cells (in which tight receptor-G protein coupling is maintained) and a comparison with the loosely coupled synaptic membrane system in which the G-protein antagonist GDPβS serves as a partial agonist have led to this theory (Rasenick et al. 1988). Consistent with the above hypothesis, Woon et al. (1989) have constructed a chimeric G protein (containing the first 356 amino acid residues of Gs and the final 36 residues of Gi at the carboxyl terminal) that they have expressed in Chinese hamster ovary (CHO) cells. This protein was unable to couple to the receptor, but the ability of this G chimera to stimulate adenylyl cyclase was quite high (in fact, it may have engaged in constitutive activation of that enzyme). Thus, if a G protein is freed from the constraints of receptor coupling, it would be expected to interact more successfully with the appropriate intracellular effector molecule. Thus, down-regulation of a Gs-linked receptor might result in increased adenylyl cyclase activity within the affected neuron by increasing receptor-independent activation of that enzyme, causing increased coupling between Gs and the adenylyl cyclase catalytic moiety. A similar phenomenon may occur in the effects of chronic antidepressant treatment on the dopamine 1 receptor-adenylyl cyclase system (De Montis et al. 1990).

What is the physiological meaning of the reconciliation of receptor-G protein-effector regulation on the action of antidepressants? The possibility of intracellular (receptor-independent) activation of neuronal adenylyl cyclase has been proposed previously. Much of the rationale for such endogenous regulation resides in the fact that, in the mammalian brain, the quantity of neurotransmitters capable of stimulating adenylyl cyclase is at least 100-fold lower than the quantity of neurotransmitters capable of inhibiting that enzyme. The current paradigms explaining the dual regulation of adenylyl cyclase require inhibition of a stimulated enzyme. Thus, neurotransmitters that act by inhibiting adenylyl cyclase might be expected to be ineffective without prior exposure of a cell to a stimulatory agonist. Intraneuronal activation of adenylyl cyclase could obviate this dilemma. A schematic illustration summarizing the action of antidepressants on the receptor-G protein-effector system is shown in Fig. 2.

Postmortem Study in Affective Disorders

Our previous study (Ozawa et al. 1993) reported that the amounts of various G-protein subunits in postmortem brain samples from the parietal and temporal cortices were the same in controls and in patients with depression, as demonstrated by immunoblotting. However, photoaffinity GTP labeling of Gi/oα, but not Gsα, was significantly increased in both cortical regions of patients with depression. In addition to basal activity, guanine nucleotide-, forskolin-, and manganese-stimulated adenylyl cyclase activities were reduced. Furthermore, an increase of phosphodieseterase binding sites (PDE type 4) was observed, suggesting that degradation of cyclic AMP is enhanced in depressed and suicidal people. Cowburn et al. (1994) found that the brains of people with depressive symptoms who had committed suicide had significant decreases in basal adenylyl cyclase activity and in guanine nucleotide-, forskolin-, and manganese-stimulated adenylyl cyclase activities to the same extent, in spite of

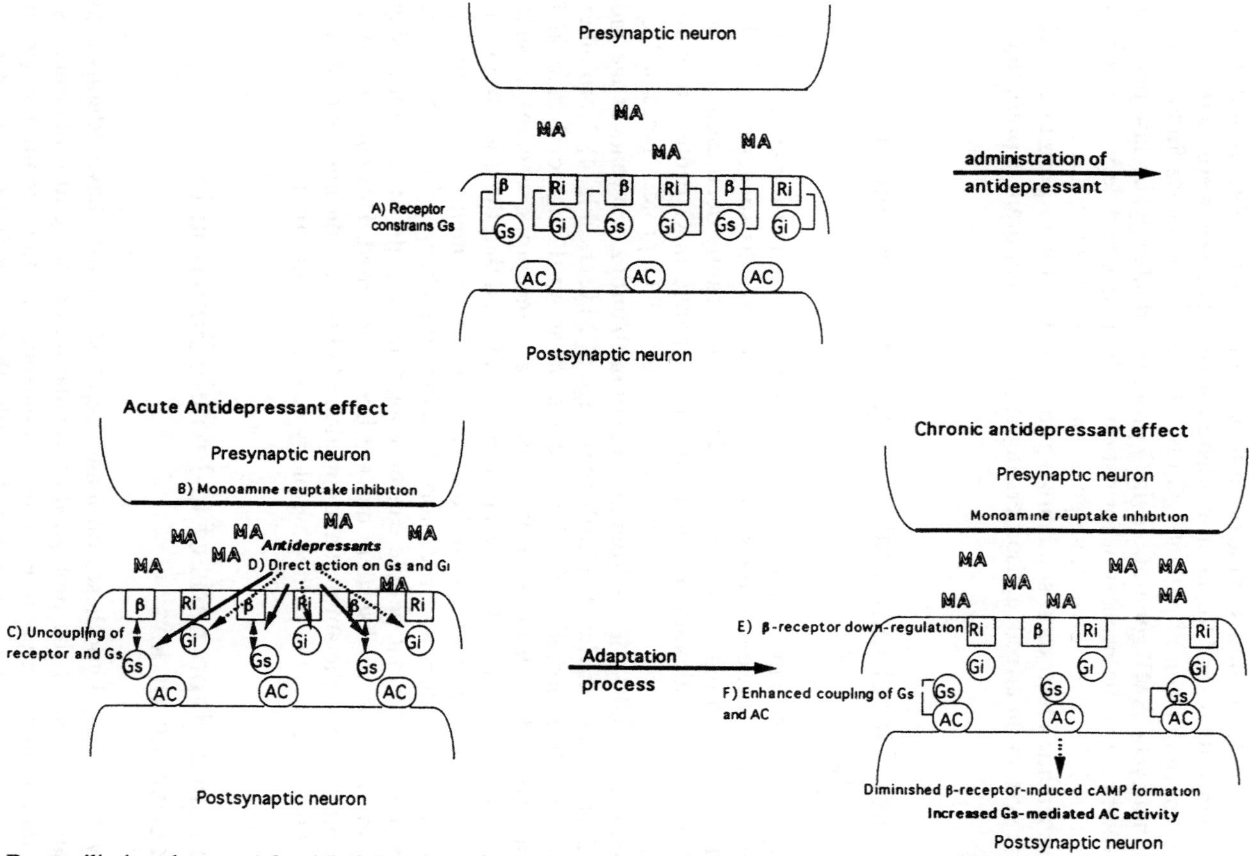

FIG. 2. Reconciliation theory. *AC*, adenylyl cyclase; *β*, β-receptor; *MA*, monoamine; R_i, Gi coupled receptor

an increase in Gs immunoreactivity. This finding agreed with the results of our study on unipolar depressive disorders, indicating the diminishing function of Gs and adenylyl cyclase or the enhancing function of Gi in the brains of patients with depression. On the other hand, Young et al. (1993) reported that the amounts of Gs- and forskolin-mediated adenylyl cyclase were increased in the postmortem brain of patients with bipolar disorders. These findings indicated that cyclic AMP generation via G protein and adenylyl cyclase plays an important role in the process of formation of the manic and depressive states and in the difference between unipolar and bipolar affective disorders.

A schematic illustration summarizing the effect of the G protein-adenylyl cyclase system on affective disorders in the postmortem brain is presented in Fig. 3.

Postnatal Developmental Changes of G Protein in Human Brains

Young et al. (1991) examined the amount of G protein in the parietal cortex of people aged between 3 days and 92 years; the results suggested that the amount of Gi and high-molecular-weight Gs significantly decreased with aging. We also investigated the developmental change in G protein in more detail. We found that the quality and quantity of G protein increased by approximately 200%–400% from the time of birth until 2 or 3 years of age and then decreased to the level at birth by the age of 10 years (Fig. 4). Kornhuber et al. (1989a,b) reported a transient increase at about the age of 2 years and then a gradual decrease of neurotransmitters and receptors, whereas no such trend was observed for MAO. Thus it can be inferred that there is a transient peak at about 2 years of age in the postreceptor components, similar to that for neurotransmitters and receptors. Whether the changes in the brains of depressed and suicidal people can be considered a state or a predisposing condition in affective disorders has not been confirmed. However, the dramatic alteration in the amount and function of G protein during the postnatal period might reflect the pathophysiology of affective disorders.

Imbalance Hypothesis of G-Protein Function in Affective Disorders

Many of the past hypotheses on manic-depressive illness have attemped to explain the cause of the biological dysregulation of the central nervous system that controls human emotion. Imbalances in the second-messenger system have been hypothesized in the pathophysiology of affective disorders (Wachtel 1989, 1990). The lack of balance in the second-messenger signaling of affective disorders has suggested that affective disorders may be caused by

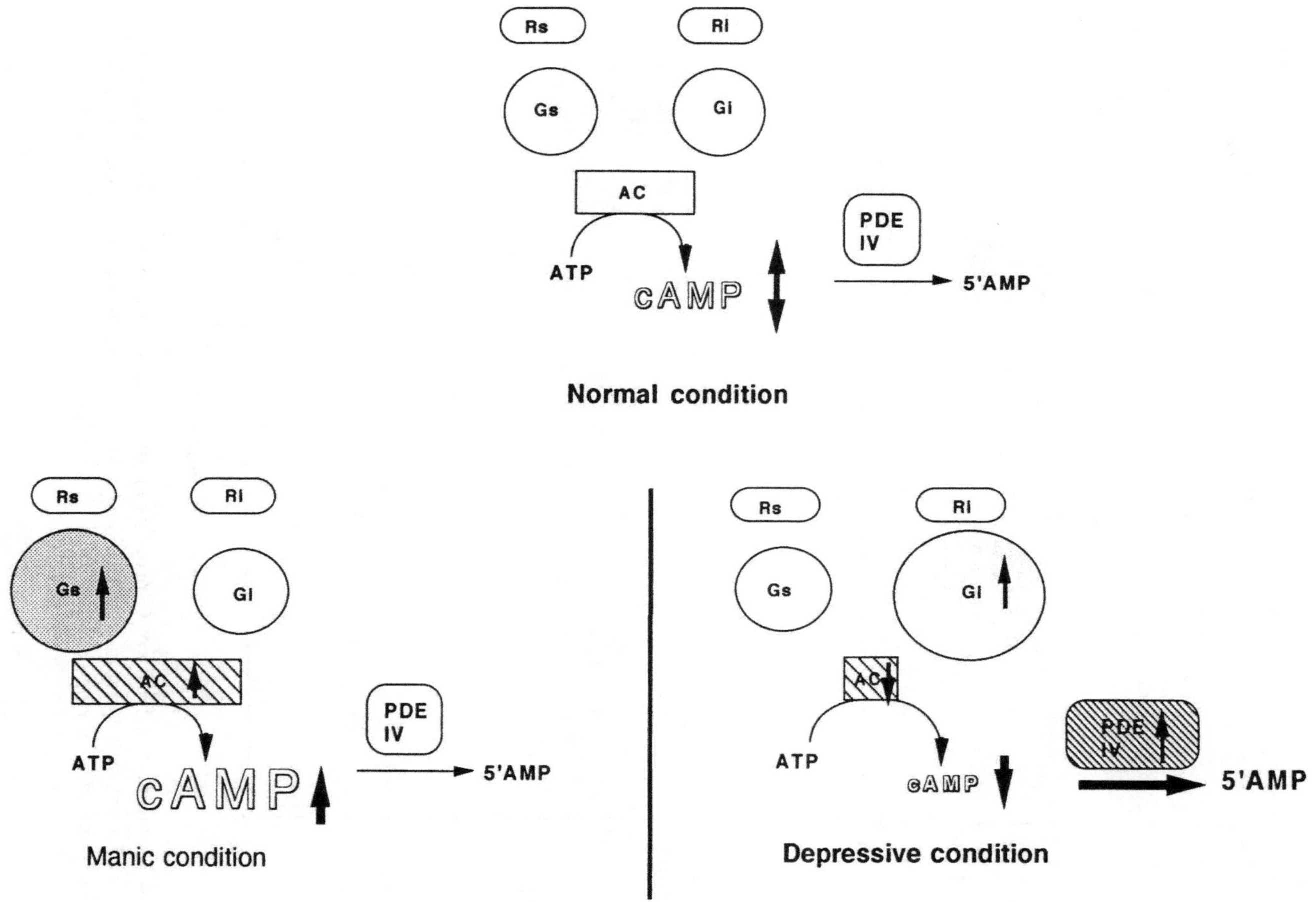

FIG. 3. cAMP production and degradation cascade. *AC*, adenylyl cyclase; *PDE IV*, phosphodiesterase type IV; R_i, Gi coupled receptor; R_s Gs coupled receptor

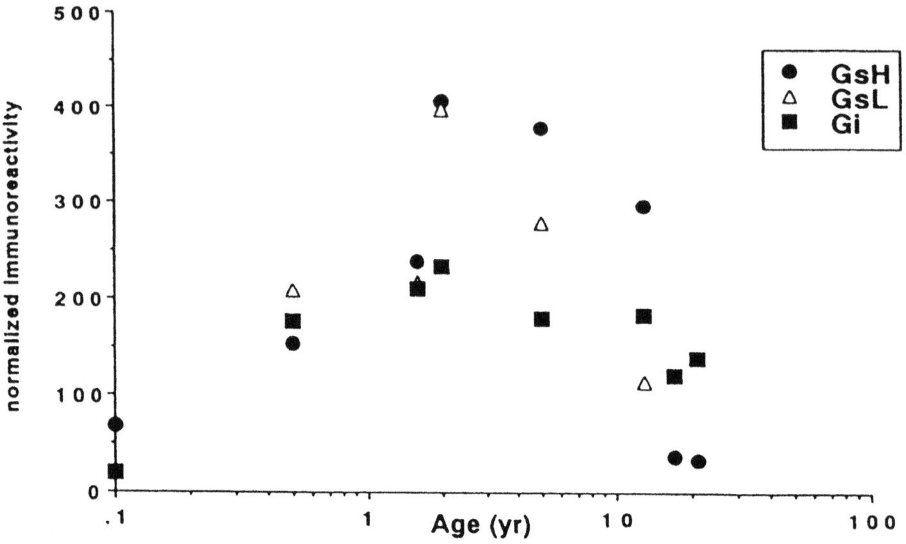

a

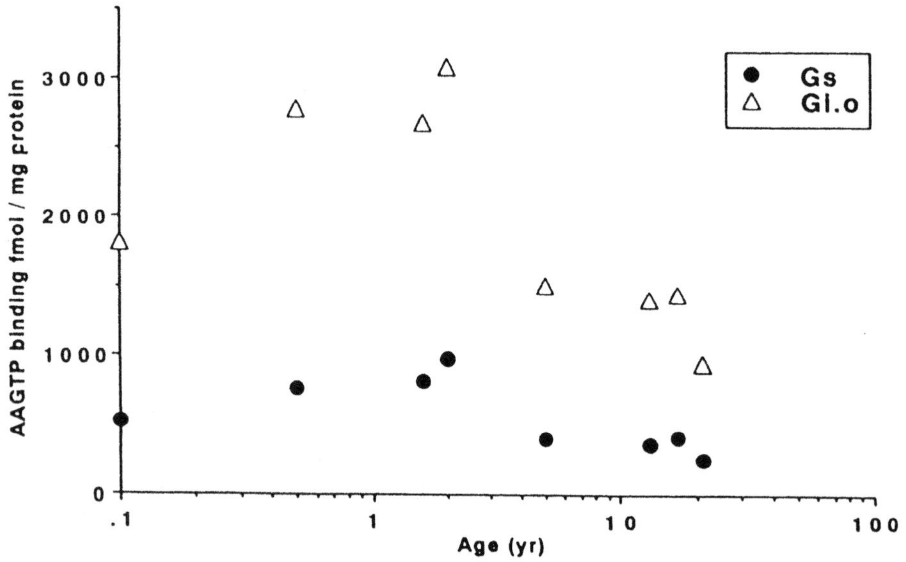

b

FIG. 4. **a** Immunoreactivity of G proteins in human cortex membrane during the early postnatal period. **b** Guanine nucleotide (AAGTP) binding of G proteins in human cortex membrane during the early postnatal period a functional disproportion of the two major second-messenger systems, with depression resulting from hypofunction of adenylyl cyclase pathways with absolute or relative dominance of the phospholipase C (PLC) pathways, and mania resulting from contrasting conditions, hypothesized from the mechanisms of action of therapeutic agents and peripheral tissue studies in affective disorders (Wachtel 1989, 1990).

On the basis of pharmacological and human brain studies by our group and others, we proposed the imbalance hypothesis of G-protein function in affective disorders (Fig. 5). Adenylyl cyclase is regulated by the balance between Gs and Gi functions. In addition, Gi- and Go-like proteins, which are ADP-ribosylated substrates of pertussis toxin, are presumed to activate the PLC system, since this toxin affects phosphoinositide metabolism. Therefore, our results indicate that a state occurring during hypofunction of the adenylyl cyclase system and hyperfunction of the PLC system through altered equilibrium of G-protein functions was observed in the proportions of Gs and Gi/o in depressed patients. Antidepressants may enhance Gs function to normalize this imbalance. Since lithium has the potency to inhibit Gs as well as Gi (Avissar and Schreiber 1992), this element suppresses both the manic and the depressive states. On the other hand, antidepressants may induce the imbalance of Gs and Gi functions because they promote Gs function rather than that of other G proteins. Consequently, this may cause depression to turn into mania and easily induce rapid cycle formation. A recent postmortem brain study of patients with bipolar affective disorders suggested that there is an imbalance between the activities of the phosphoinositide system via Gq function, which was decreased, and the adenylyl cyclase system via Gs function, which was increased, relative to matched controls (Jope et al. 1996). Enhanced postsynaptic 5-HT_{2A} receptor function in depressed patients was reported in postmortem brain and peripheral tissue (Kusumi and Koyama, this volume). Additionally, it has been reported that chronic treatment with several antidepressants and selective serotonin reuptake inhibitors (SSRIs) is able to induce down-regulation of 5-HT_{2A} receptor function. Thus, we speculate that the proportions of Gs and Gi/o are altered in the manic state, a state occurring during hyperfunction of the adenylyl cyclase system and hypofunction of the PLC system via 5-HT_{2A} receptors.

This hypothesis is based on the facilitation of Gi function in depressive and manic conditions. In the mammalian brain, there is 10 times more Gi (which inhibits the function of adenylyl cyclase) than Gs (which stimulates the function of the enzyme). Our preliminary data suggest that the NaF-mediated inhibitory effect on adenylyl cyclase is stronger than the activation effect in the human cerebral cortex compared with that in rats. As G-protein levels change in the developmental period, persons who have a predisposition for dominance of Gi function over that of Gs may be affected by some environmental or constitutional impacts of critical duration. For such persons, there may be a trend toward altered equilibrium of G-protein function, and they may suffer from affective disorders caused by emotional stress.

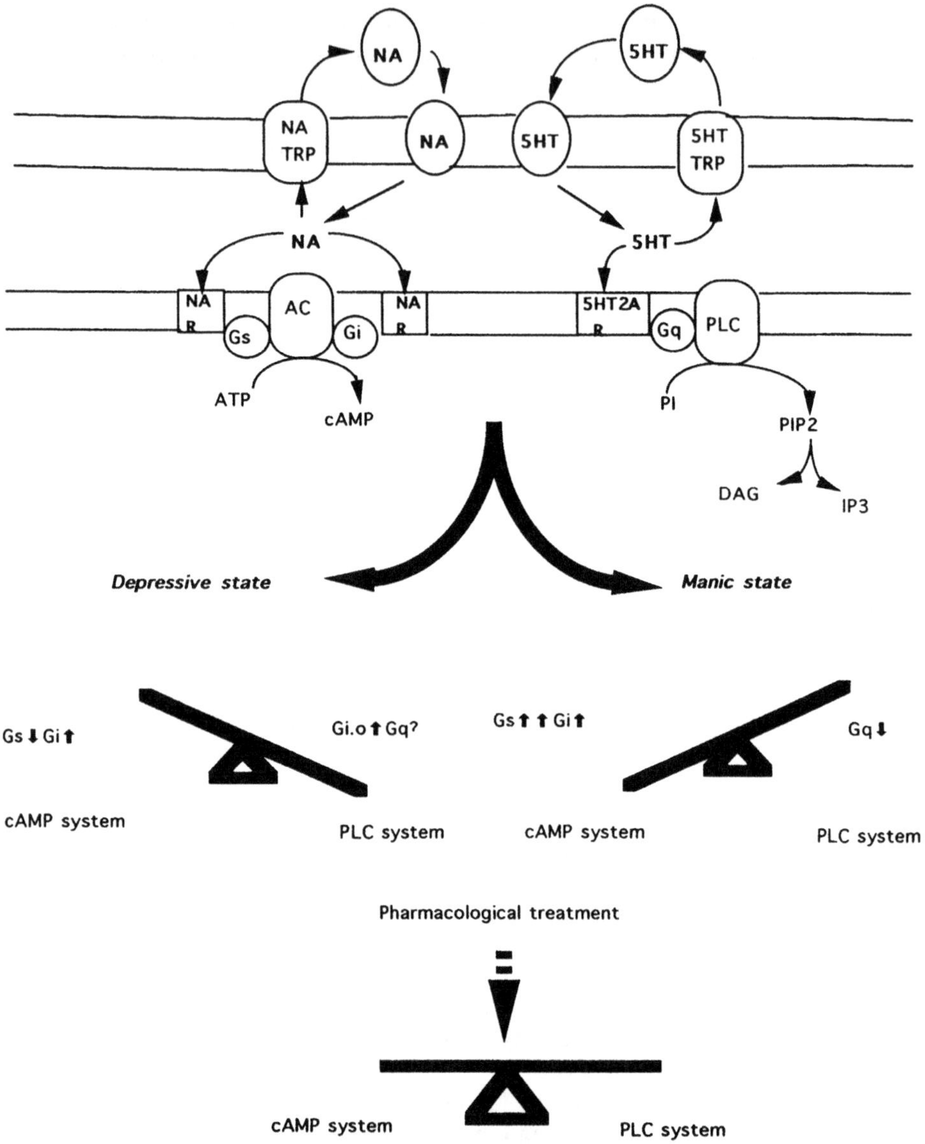

Fig. 5. G-protein function imbalance theory of affective disorders. *AC*, adenylyl cyclase; *DAG*, diacylglycerol; *IP*$_3$, inositol 1,4,5-trisphosphate; *NA*, noradrenaline; *PI*, phosphatidylinositol; *PIP*$_2$, phosphatidylinositol 4,5-bisphosphate; *PLC*, phospholipase C; *R*, receptor; *TRP*, transportor

Selectivity of Treatment Drugs in the Light of Signal Transduction

There is some evidence that clomipramine and amitriptyline, which are 5-HT reuptake inhibitors despite also being tricyclics, are effective in quelling sadness and psychomotor agitation. In contrast, desipramine, which is a selective noradrenaline reuptake inhibitor, ameliorates psychomotor retardation. Thus, the selection of drug treatment must take into consideration the varieties of neural transmission. On the other hand, in the near future, we should consider not only the side stream of signaling but also the upstream and downstream signaling in the selection of drug treatment (Fig. 6).

Rolipram is a novel dialkoxyphenyl pyrrolidone derivative that inhibits Ca/calmodulin-independent cyclic AMP phosphodiesterase activity, inducing an increase in cyclic AMP content. This compound had antidepressive activity in a clinical study (Horowski et al. 1985). Forskolin was also shown to be predictive of antidepressive effects in animal models because of enhanced availability of cyclic AMP brain effector cells (Wachtel and Loshmann 1986; Maeda et al. 1996). Basic and clinical trials of inositol (a second-messenger precursor) for affective disorders and other neuropsychiatric diseases are now in progress

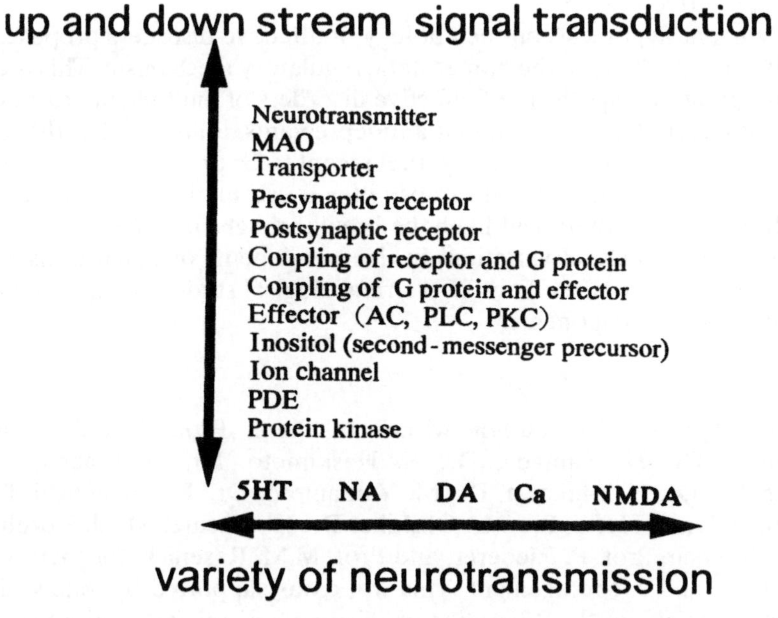

FIG. 6. Selectivity of treatment drugs for vertical and horizontal streams of signaling. *AC*, adenylyl cyclase; *DA*, dopamine; *NA*, noradrenaline; *NMDA*, *N*-methyl-D-aspartate; *MAO*, monoamine oxidase; *PDE*, phosphodiesterase; *PKC*, protein kinase C; *PLC*, phospholipase C

(Belmaker et al. 1995). Additionally, to consider one alternative treatment, methyl-vitamin B_{12} (mecobalamin), a methyl donor involved in the synthesis of S-adenosyl-L-methionine, has clinical effects on peripheral nerve disorders as well as central nerve disorders (delayed sleep syndrome and seasonal affective disorders). Our preliminary study suggested that mecobalamin has direct effects on the enhancement of AC activity via alteration of coupling between G protein AC molecules rather than activation of the molecules themselves.

Conclusion

The classical research on the actions of antidepressants and the pathology of affective disorders has been based on the question of whether there are increases or decreases of neuronal signal transduction in specific brain regions. In terms of the actions of antidepressants, prolonged treatment seems to be essential to obtain clinical and neurochemical effects, suggesting that these actions involve some adaptive neurochemical mechanisms. Antidepressants have effects on multiple neurotransmitters, including noradrenaline, 5-HT, dopamine, $GABA_B$, acetylcholine, and neuropeptides, alone or in combination. Thus, a single neurotransmitter is unlikely to be responsible for all the actions of antidepressants.

The current hypothesis on the etiology of affective disorders proposes that there is some problem in the homeostatic regulatory mechanism. This is called the dysregulation hypothesis of affective disorders of multiple neurotransmitters. It has been demonstrated that antidepressants, lithium, other drugs, and electroconvulsive therapy modify the receptor-G protein-effector system, causing reorchestration of neurotransmitter dysregulation in affective disorders. In the future, there will likely be breakthroughs in genetic research on some primary structural variations in the components of signal transduction (G proteins, effectors, etc.) and in pharmacological studies on agents that act directly on such components.

Acknowledgments. The author wishes to thank Prof. T. Saito, Dr. Y. Katamura, Dr. H. Kamada, Dr. E. Hashimoto, Dr. H. Maeda, Dr. S. Shichinohe, Dr. H. Ishikawa, Dr. M. Yamamoto, Dr. T. Yamaguchi, Dr. N. Amemiya, Dr. S. Hatta, Prof. H. Ohshika, Dr. H. Wachtel, Dr. J. Kornhuber, Dr. L. Froelich, Prof. P. Riederer, and Prof. M.M. Rasenick, for their helpful suggestions and encouragement. This work was supported by fellowships of the Japan Society for the Promotion of Sciences for Japanese Junior Scientists, the Scientific Research Fund of the Ministry of Education, Science, and Culture of Japan, and grants on affective disorders and brain science from the Ministry of Health and Welfare of Japan.

References

Avissar S, Schreiber G (1992) The involvement of guanine nucleotide binding proteins in the pathogenesis and treatment of affective disorders. Biol Psychiatr 31:435–459

Belmaker RH, Bersudsky Y, Benjamin J, Agam G, Levine J, Kofman O (1995) Manipulation of inositol-linked second messenger systems as a therapeutic strategy in psychiatry. Adv Biochem Psychopharmacol 49:67–84

Cheung J, Rasenick MM (1995) Chronic antidepressant treatment facilitates G protein activation without altering G protein content. J Pharmacol Exp Ther 275:509–517

Cowburn RF, Marcusson JO, Eriksson A, Wiehanger B, O'Neill C (1994) Adenylyl cyclase activity and G-protein subunit levels in postmortem frontal cortex of suicide victims. Brain Res 633:297–304

De Montis GM, Devoto P, Gessa GL (1990) Selective adenylyl cyclase increase in the limbic area of long-term imipramine-treated rats. Eur J Pharmacol 180:169–174

Dibner MD, Molinoff PB (1979) Agonist-induced changes in beta-adrenergic receptor density and receptor mediated responsiveness in slices of rat cerebral cortex. J Pharmacol Exp Ther 210:433–439

Duman RS, Strada SJ, Enna SJ (1985) Effect of imipramine and adrenocorticotropin administration on the rat brain norepinephrine-coupled cyclic nucleotide generating system: alterations in alpha and beta adrenergic components. J Pharmacol Exp Ther 234:409–414

Hancock AA, Marsh CL (1984) Selective down-regulation of high agonist affinity beta adrenergic receptors following chronic desipramine treatment. Fed Proc 43:873

Horowski R, Sastre-Y-Hernandez M (1985) Clinical effects of the neurotropic selective cAMP phosphodiesterase inhibitor rolipram in depressed patients. Global evaluation of the preliminary reports. Curr Ther Res 38:23–29

Jope RS, Song L, Li PP, Young LT, Kish SJ, Pacheco MA, Warsh JJ (1996) The phosphoinositide signal transduction system is impaired in bipolar affective disorder brain. J Neurochem 66:2401–2409

Kamada H, Ozawa H, Saito T, Hatta S, Takahata N (1997) Dimeric tubulin-stimulated adenylyl cyclase activity is augmented after long-term amitriptyline treatment. Life Sci 60:57–66

Kornhuber J, Konradi C, Mack-Burkhardt F, Riederer P, Heinsen H, Beckmann H (1989a) Ontogenesis of monoamine oxidase-A and -B in the human brain frontal cortex. Brain Res 499:81–86

Kornhuber J, Retz W, Riederer P (1989b) Effect of antemortem and postmortem factors on [^{3}H]glutamate binding in the human brain. Life Sci 45:312–317

Lesch KP, Aulakh CS, Tolliver TJ, Hill JL, Murphy DL (1991) Regulation of G proteins by chronic antidepressant drug treatment in rat brain: tricyclics but not clorgyline increase G$o\alpha$ subunits. Eur J Pharmacol 207:361–364

Maeda H, Ozawa H, Amemiya N, Kaneta K, Saito T, Takahata N (1996) Effects Of forskolin administration on behavioral response to forced swimming in the rat. Neurosci Abst 22:374

McLaughlin M, Ross BM, Milligan G, McCulloch J, Knowler JT (1991) Robustness of G proteins in Alzheimer's disease: an immunoblot study. J Neurochem 57:9–14

Menkes DB, Rasenick MM, Wheeler M, Bitensky MW (1983) Guanosine triphosphate activation of brain adenylyl cyclase: Enhancement by long-term antidepressant treatment. Science 129:65–67

Mishra R, Janowsky A , Sulser F (1980) Action of mianserin and zimelidine on the norepinephrine receptor coupled adenylyl cyclase system in brain: subsensitivity without reduction in beta-adrenergic receptor binding. Neuropharmacology 19:983–987

Newman ME, Lerer B (1989) Post-receptor increases in adenylyl cyclase activity after chronic antidepressant treatment: relationship to receptor desensitization. Eur J Pharmacol 162:345–352

O'Donnell JM, Frazer A (1985) Effects of clenbuterol and antidepressant drugs on beta adrenergic receptor N-protein coupling in cerebral cortex of the rat. J Pharmacol Exp Ther 234:30–36

Okada F, Tokumitsu Y, Ui M (1986) Desensitization of beta-adrenergic receptor-coupled adenylyl cyclase in cerebral cortex after in vivo treatment of rats with desipramine. J Neurochem 47:454–459

Ozawa H, Rasenick MM (1989) Coupling of the stimulatory GTP-binding protein, Gs, to rat synaptic membrane adenylate cyclase is enhanced subsequent to chronic antidepressant treatment. Mol Pharmcol 36:803–808

Ozawa H, Rasenick MM (1991) Chronic electroconvulsive treatment augments coupling of the GTP-binding protein Gs to the catalytic moiety of adenylyl cyclase in a manner similar to that seen with chronic antidepressant drugs. J Neurochem 56:330–338

Ozawa H, Gsell W, Froelich L, Beckmann H, Riederer P (1993) Imbalance of the Gs and Gi/o function in post-mortem human brain of depressed patients. J Neural Transm [GenSect]94:63–69

Ozawa H, Katamura Y, Hatta S, Amemiya N, Saito T, Ohshika H, Takahata N (1994) Antidepressants directly influence in situ binding of guanine nucleotide in synaptic membrane. Life Sci 54:925–932

Rasenick MM, Hughes JM, Wang N (1988) Guanosine-5'-o-thiodiphosphate functions as a partial agonist for the receptor-independent stimulation of neural adenylate cyclase. Brain Res 488:105–113

Seeman KB (1987) Forskolin and adenylyl cyclase. ISI Atlas Pharmacol 1:250–253

Simon M, Strathman M, Gautam N (1991) Diversity of G proteins in signal transduction. Science 252:802–808

Tiong AHK, Richardson JS (1990) Beta-adrenoceptor and post-receptor components show different rates of desensitization to desipramine. Eur J Pharmacol 188:411–415

Wachtel H (1989) Dysbalance of neuronal second messenger function in aetiology of affective disorders; a pathophysiological concept hypothesizing defects beyond first messenger receptors. J Neural Transm 75:21–29

Wachtel H (1990) The second-messenger dysbalance hypothesis of affective disorders. Pharmacopsychiatry 23:27–32

Wachtel H, Loshmann PA (1986) Effects of forskolin and cyclic nucleotides in animal models predictive of antidepressive activity: interaction with rolipram. Psychopharmacology 90:430–435

Woon CW, Soparkar S, Heasley L, Johnson GL (1989) Expression of a Gαs/Gαi chimera that constitutively activates cAMP synthesis. J Biol Chem 264:5687–5693

Yamamoto H, Tomita U, Mikuni M, Kobayashi I, Kagaya A, Katada T, Ui M, Takahashi K (1992) Direct activation of purified Go-type GTP binding protein by tricyclic antidepressants. Neurosci Lett 139:194–196

Young LT, Warsh JJ, Li PP, Siu KP, Becker L, Gilbert J, Hornykiewicz O, Kish SJ (1991) Maturation and aging effects on guanine nucleotide binding protein immunoreactivity in human brain. Dev Brain Res 61:243–248
Young LT, Li PP, Kish SJ, Siu KP, Kamble A, Hornykiewicz O, Warsh JJ (1993) Cerebral cortex Gsα protein levels and forskolin-stimulated cyclic AMP formation are increased in bipolar affective disorders. J Neurochem 61:890–898

Protein Phosphorylation System in the Mechanism of Action of Antidepressants

S. MIYAMOTO and M. ASAKURA

Introduction

Although antidepressants are currently in widespread use as psychotropic drugs, their precise mechanism of action has not yet been elucidated. The strong potency of antidepressants for inhibiting the reuptake of catecholamines into presynaptic nerve terminals was initially the basis for Schildkraut's proposal of the monoaminergic hypothesis of affective disorders (Schildkraut 1965). This hypothesis should be extended or revised, as the inhibition of catecholamine reuptake is observed within minutes to hours after administration of a single antidepressant, whereas the clinical effect in depressive patients is often seen only after 1 to 3 weeks of daily treatment. Vetulani and Sulser (1975) proposed that this delay in the occurrence of the therapeutic action could be correlated with the development of noradrenergic subsensitivity of the cyclic adenosine monophosphate (cAMP) generating system in the brain after chronic, but not acute, treatment with tricyclic antidepressants and with some atypical antidepressants.

During the 1980s particular attention was focused on defining long-term modifications in the sensitivity of presynaptic and postsynaptic receptors following prolonged antidepressant treatment. A number of receptor-binding studies have indicated that long-term, but not short-term, treatment with clinically effective antidepressants commonly results in a decrease in β-adrenergic and serotonin-2 (5-hydroxy tryptamine, 5-HT) receptor binding in the rat cerebral cortex (Peroutka and Snyder 1980; Charney et al. 1981). These receptor changes represent only the first step in the cascade of signal transduction pathways involved in the action of antidepressants. For revealing functional changes in neurons, studies at the level of receptors have limited value. In addition, most of the newer antidepressants, such as the selective 5-HT reuptake inhibitors and the specific serotonin and norepinephrine (NE)

Department of Neuropsychiatry, St. Marianna University School of Medicine, 2-16-1 Sugao, Miyamae-ku, Kawasaki, Kanagawa 216, Japan reuptake inhibitors, have not been shown to consistently alter the number of β-adrenergic and 5-HT-2 receptors in the rat cerebral cortex.

Therefore, more recent studies have been focused on neuronal signal transduction processes beyond the level of receptors as potential target sites for the action of antidepressants. It has been demonstrated that long-term treatment with antidepressants leads to neuronal adaptive changes and modifications in the function of receptor-coupled guanosine triphosphate (GTP, or G)-binding proteins (Ozawa and Rasenick 1989), in the action of protein kinases and phosphoproteins (Nestler et al. 1989; Perez et al. 1989, 1991; Brunello et al. 1990; Racagni et al. 1992; Mann et al. 1995), and in the regulation of gene expression at the nuclear level (Morinobu et al. 1995; Nibuya et al. 1996).

In this review, we summarize the results of recent studies and our observations on the protein phosphorylation systems, particularly on the cAMP-dependent phosphorylation system, which may be involved in the mechanism of action of antidepressants. Furthermore, possible implications of the involvement of specific phosphoproteins in the biochemical effects of antidepressant drugs are discussed.

Protein Phosphorylation Systems

Protein phosphorylation appears to represent one, possibly the most important, molecular mechanism by which extracellular signals produce their biological responses in specific target neurons (Walaas and Greengard 1991). Chemical transmitters are released at synapses and stimulate respective receptors at postsynaptic membranes in the nervous system. When the nerve impulses reach the nerve endings and neurotransmitters are released at synapses, signal transduction occurs at the plasma membranes. Consequently, the levels of the second messengers such as cAMP, cyclic guanosine monophosphate (cGMP), calcium, diacylglycerol, and inositol triphosphate increase in the nerve cells. The target substances for these active compounds may be protein kinases. Therefore the actions of the second messengers may be mediated through the activation of protein kinases (Fig. 1).

Protein kinases are phosphotransferases that catalyze the transfer of phosphate from ATP, or sometimes GTP, to specific serine, threonine, or tyrosine residues in substrate proteins. There are many second messenger dependent and independent protein kinases in the brain, they are classified into serine/threonine kinases, tyrosine kinases, and serine/threonine/tyrosine kinases (Girault 1993). Protein kinases differ in size, subunit structure, distribution in brain, subcellular localization, regulation of activation, and substrate specificity. More than 70 phosphoproteins are found in the brain, including enzymes involved in neurotransmitter biosynthesis, synaptic vesicle-associated proteins, protein phosphatase inhibitors, neurotransmitter receptors, ion channels, ion transporters, cytoskeletal proteins, and transcription factors, all of which appear to be particularly important in neuronal function (Nestler et al. 1984).

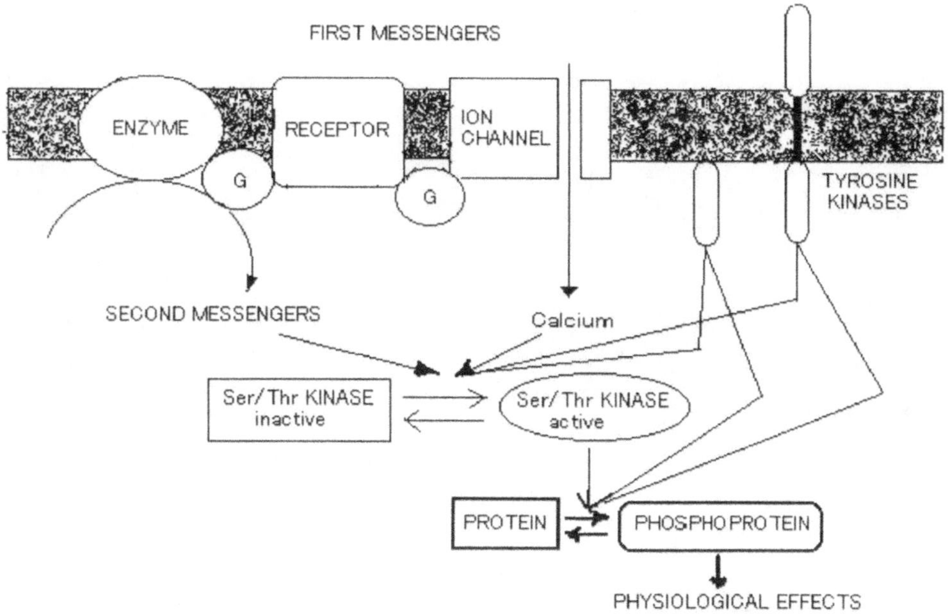

FIG. 1. Some pathways by which extracellular signals alter protein phosphorylation in neurons. (Adapted from Girault, 1993)

Processes that are reversibly controlled by protein phosphorylation require not only a protein kinase but also a protein phosphatase. The phosphoprotein phosphatases dephosphorylate the phosphoproteins, thereby returning the particular protein phosphorylation system to its basal state. Phosphorylation levels of substrate proteins can be increased by activation of protein kinases, inhibition of protein phosphatases, or changes in the properties of the proteins themselves as targets for different kinases or phosphatases (Walaas and Greengard 1991). Some substrate proteins are phosphorylated by multiple protein kinases and consequently exhibit common functional responses in the nervous system. Protein phosphorylation systems allow not only the transduction of extracellular signals into biochemical reactions inside the nerve cell but also the "computation or amplification" of distinct extracellular signals and their "convergence or integration" over time (Girault 1993).

cAMP-Dependent Phosphorylation System

Binding of an agonist to the stimulatory or inhibitory receptor transmits a signal via the stimulatory or inhibitory G proteins to the catalytic subunit, resulting in activation or inactivation of adenylate cyclase. Activation of ade-

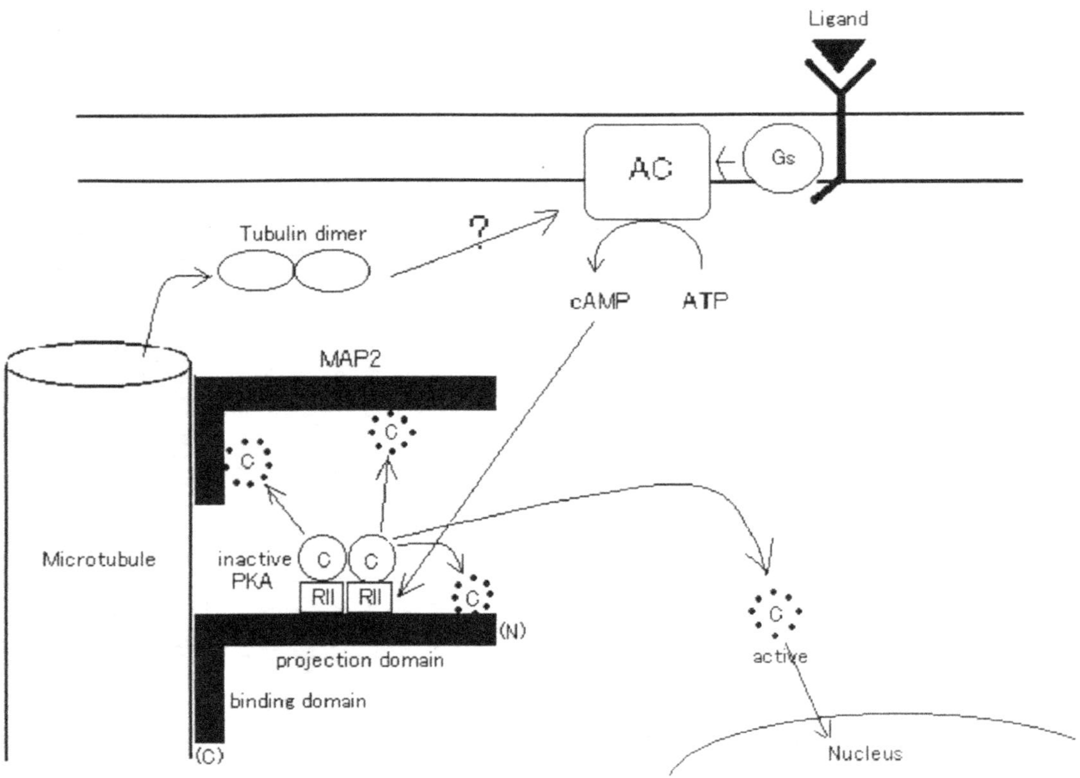

FIG. 2. MAP2–PKA complex. MAP2 projections are shown distributed on the microtubule surface. The NH_2-terminal of MAP2 contains a binding domain for the RII regulatory subunit of PKA. PKA is a tetramer composed of two cAMP-binding regulatory subunits and two catalytic subunits (*C*). Upon cAMP binding to RII, the active catalytic subunits are released from the MAP2-R_2 complex and are free to phosphorylate MAP2. The phosphorylation of MAP2 by PKA induces inhibition of microtubule assembly. *PKA*, cAMP-dependent protein kinase; *MAP2*, microtubule-associated protein 2; *cAMP*, cyclic adenspine monophosphate; *ATP*, adenosine triphosphate; *AC*, adenylate cyclase; *Gs*, stimulatory guanosine triphosphate-binding protein; (*N*), amino terminus; (C), carboxy terminus. (Adapted from Theurkauf and Vallee, 1982)

nylate cyclase induces hydrolysis of ATP to cAMP (Fig. 2). The second messenger cAMP exerts nearly all of its effects by activating cAMP-dependent protein kinase (PKA). PKA, first described by Walsh et al. (1968), is present at high levels in the brain and exists in two main isozymic forms. PKA is a tetrameric holoenzyme composed of two catalytic (C) subunits (40 kDa apparent molecular mass) and two regulatory (R) subunits, which form the intracellular receptor for cAMP (Nimmo and Cohen 1977). These isozymes, designated types I and II PKA, are composed of the RI (47–49 kDa) or the RII (51–55 kDa) regulatory subunit, respectively. Both isozymes are activated by binding of the newly formed intracellular cAMP to the R subunits, resulting in dissociation of the holoenzyme to a complex of two R subunits and cAMP, and to two active C subunits, which, in turn, phosphorylate specific substrate proteins (Walaas and Greengard 1991).

Effect of Antidepressant Treatment on the PKA System

It has been well documented that chronic treatment with antidepressants reduces the responsiveness of the norepinephrine (NE)-β-adrenoceptor-coupled adenylate cyclase system in the rat brain (Charney et al. 1981). A role for the PKA system in the long-term effects of antidepressant treatment was initially reported by Moyer et al. (1986). They found that repeated treatment with desipramine (10 mg/kg IP for 5 days), a tricyclic antidepressant, but not with other antidepressants such as zimelidine, iprindole, or fluoxetine, caused a significant decrease in the cytosolic level of PKA activity in the rat pineal gland. They also found that isoproterenol-induced activation of PKA was reduced by repeated desipramine treatment. Based on their results, these authors speculated that the rate of PKA synthesis was decreased or that PKA was translocated from the soluble to the particulate fraction of the rat pineal gland after repeated administration of desipramine. They did not observe any changes in PKA activity in the particulate fractions. Moreover, this effect of desipramine on PKA was limited to specific brain regions such as the pineal gland.

Nestler et al. (1989) subsequently found evidence to support PKA as a target site of therapeutic antidepressant action. They showed that chronic, but not acute, administration of imipramine (15 mg/kg IP for 18 days) or tranylcypromine (7.5 mg/kg IP for 18 days) resulted in a decrease in PKA activity in soluble fractions of the rat frontal cortex but an increase in PKA activity in the crude nuclear fraction. These authors speculated that chronic antidepressant treatment might stimulate the translocation of PKA from the cytosol to the nucleus and result in the phosphorylation of specific nuclear proteins, which would then lead to changes in gene expression. Extending this observation, Melia et al. (1992) found that chronic administration of imipramine (15 mg/kg IP for 18 days) resulted in a significant decrease in the level of soluble PKA activity in the locus ceruleus, the major noradrenergic nucleus in brain. In this brain region, the level of PKA in the particulate fraction was not significantly influenced by imipramine treatment. It is therefore conceivable that antidepressant-induced increases in nuclear PKA activity represent a region-specific effect.

A report by Nibuya et al. (1996) has provided much stronger support for the hypothesis that the cAMP–PKA-gene expression cascade is a common target of various types of antidepressant drugs. They focused on the expression of the nuclear transcription factor, the cAMP response element binding protein (CREB). In the case of the cAMP pathway, the activated catalytic subunit of PKA is translocated to the nucleus and phosphorylates CREB at serine 133 (Hagiwara et al. 1993). Nibuya et al. (1996) reported that long-term treatment with any of several classes of antidepressants, such as desipramine (15 mg/kg), imipramine (15 mg/kg), tranylcypromine (7.5 mg/kg), sertraline (10 mg/kg), or fluoxetine (5 mg/kg), resulted in a significant increase in the level of CREB mRNA in the rat hippocampus. It is noteworthy that although desensitization of certain NE and 5-HT receptors is often observed after chronic administration of antidepressants, the functional output of these receptor-coupled intracellular cascades involved in the expression of CREB is up-regulated, not down-regulated. However, little is known about the cytosolic changes in PKA regulation and in substrate proteins for PKA that are induced by chronic antidepressant treatment.

Perez et al. (1989) highlighted the potential involvement of the cAMP-binding proteins in the cytosolic fraction of the rat cerebral cortex in the mechanism of action of antidepressants. They found that chronic, but not acute, administration of desipramine (10 mg/kg IP for 15 days) induced an increase in the covalent binding of 8-azido-[^{32}P]cAMP to the 52-kDa protein (RII regulatory subunit of PKA) but not to the 47-kDa protein (RI regulatory subunit of PKA) in both soluble and crude microtubule fractions of the rat cerebral cortex. Furthermore, these authors reported that long-term treatment with different antidepressants, such as fluoxetine (10 mg/kg IP for 10 days) or the (+) isomer of oxaprotiline (10 mg/kg IP for 10 days), which specifically inhibit 5-HT and NE reuptake, respectively, resulted in increased photoactivated incorporation of 8-azido-[^{32}P]cAMP only into the 52-kDa cAMP receptor in both soluble and crude microtubule fractions of the rat cerebral cortex (Perez et al. 1991). These results suggest that chronic antidepressant treatment induces an increase in the amount of the RII regulatory subunit of PKA associated with the crude microtubule fraction, and that RII is a common intracellular target site of various classes of antidepressants. The precise mechanism underlying the increase in the amount of the RII subunit and its functional role remain to be elucidated. It is therefore important to study the changes in phosphorylation of specific proteins that are substrates for PKA in the cytosol in response to chronic antidepressant treatment.

Effect of Antidepressant Treatment on Phosphorylation of Substrate Proteins for PKA

A pioneering work with respect to the phosphorylation, after antidepressant treatment, of substrate proteins for protein kinases was reported by Perez et al. (1989). They paid particular attention to the cytoskeletal protein microtubule-associated protein 2 (MAP2). Among the neuronal cytoskeletal proteins, MAP2 has the unique properties of its subcellular localization. The high-molecular-weight form of MAP2 is present at high concentrations in dendrites (neuronal structures specialized to receive the synaptic input), where it appears in association with microtubules (see Johnson and Jope 1992 for review). MAP2, a high-molecular-weight protein (280–300 kDa), was originally found to be a substrate for PKA (Sloboda et al. 1975), but more recent studies have shown that MAP2 can be phosphorylated at a large number of sites by a variety of other protein kinases, including calcium/calmodulin-dependent protein kinase II (CaM kinase II) (Goldenring et al. 1983; Schulman 1984), calcium/phospholipid-dependent protein kinase (PKC) (Akiyama et al. 1986), and tyrosine-specific protein kinases (Kadowaki et al. 1985). It is therefore of interest to study whether the cAMP- or calcium-dependent phosphorylation system associated with MAP2 is a postsynaptic target for the action of antidepressants.

Perez et al. (1989) reported that repeated administration of desipramine (10 mg/kg IP for 8 and 15 days) resulted in modification of the pattern of endogenous phosphorylation of a soluble cAMP-dependent phosphoprotein with molecular weight 280 kDa in both soluble and crude microtubule fractions of the rat cerebral cortex. The amount of radioactive phosphate incorporated into the 280-kDa protein band in the cerebral cortex of rats treated with desipramine was significantly higher than in control rats, under both basal and cAMP-stimulated conditions. These authors identified this 280-kDa protein as the soluble form of MAP2. It is known that approximately one-third of the total cytosolic type II PKA in the brain is bound, through RII subunits, to MAP2 (Theurkauf and Vallee 1982) (Fig. 2). Based on their findings, these investigators suggested that an increase in the amount of RII and in the rate of cAMP-dependent endogenous phosphorylation of MAP2 in the rat cerebral cortex is among the adaptive changes elicited by chronic, but not acute, treatment with desipramine (Perez et al. 1989; Brunello et al. 1990). This finding does not seem to allow a direct correlation of increased amounts of RII with effects on MAP2 phosphorylation to be convincing because changes in the activity of PKA or the protein phosphatases associated with MAP2 are unclear. Moreover, the functional output of these phenomena remains to be elucidated. It is thus of interest to examine the influence of chronic administration of antidepressants on the phosphorylation status of MAP2 in vivo as well as its physiological responses after phosphorylation.

Effect of Antidepressant Treatment on Phosphorylation of MAP2

To clarify the changes in the extent or the sites of phosphorylation of MAP2 in vivo after administration of antidepressants, we examined the phosphorylation of MAP2 by immunoblotting using several monoclonal antibodies that recognize only the specific phosphorylated amino acid residues. Adult male Wistar rats were subcutaneously administered desipramine (20 mg/kg), maprotiline (30 mg/kg), citalopram (30 mg/kg), or haloperidol (5 mg/kg) once daily for 14 days. The rats were decapitated 24 h after administration of the last dose. MAP2 was prepared from the cerebrocortical boiled supernatant fraction subsequent to immunoprecipitation of MAP2 by a method described previously (Miyamoto et al. 1995a). The immunoprecipitated MAP2 was subjected to sodium dodecyl sulfate-polyacrylamide gel electrophoresis (SDS-PAGE) and Western blotting using monoclonal antibodies such as antiphosphoserine, antiphosphothreonine, or antiphosphotyrosine antibodies.

Figure 3 shows no significant difference in the immunoreactivity of MAP2 immunoprecipitated from the cerebrocortical supernatant fraction for chronic saline (lane 1)-treated and desipramine (lane 2)-treated animals. Chronic treatment with desipramine induced a significant increase (by 43%) in the immunoreactivity of the phosphoserine residues of immunoprecipitated MAP2 when compared to the controls (Fig. 3A, lanes 3 and 4). In contrast, there was no significant increase in the immunoreactivity of phosphothreonine (Fig. 3A, lanes 5 and 6) or phosphotyrosine (Fig. 3A, lanes 7 and 8) residues of MAP2 between control and desipramine-treated rats. As shown in Fig. 4, a similar increase in the immunoreactivity of the phosphoserine residues of MAP2 was observed after long-term treatment with maprotiline (by 36%) or citalopram (by 20%) but not with haloperidol (a dopamine D2 receptor antagonist and antipsychotic agent). A single injection of desipramine, maprotiline, citalopram, or haloperidol failed to alter either the concentration or the level of phosphorylation of MAP2 in the rat cerebral cortex (Miyamoto et al. 1995a). These findings suggest that chronic, but not acute, administration of various classes of antidepressant commonly induces an increase in the phosphorylation of serine residues of MAP2 without changes in the total concentration of MAP2. The results confirm our preliminary data (Miyamoto et al. 1993), which indicate no changes in the amount of soluble MAP2 after chronic antidepressant treatment, and support the results of the phosphorylation studies by Perez et al. (1989) and Brunello et al. (1990) in which the incorporation of ^{32}P into MAP2 in vitro was investigated.

As mentioned above, MAP2 is an excellent substrate for a variety of protein kinases (Johnson and Jope 1992). It is thus possible that the increased serine phosphorylation of MAP2 observed after repeated administration of antidepressants is attributable to the increased activity of a specific serine-threonine kinase, possibly PKA, CaM kinase II, or PKC. Despite this possibility, it has

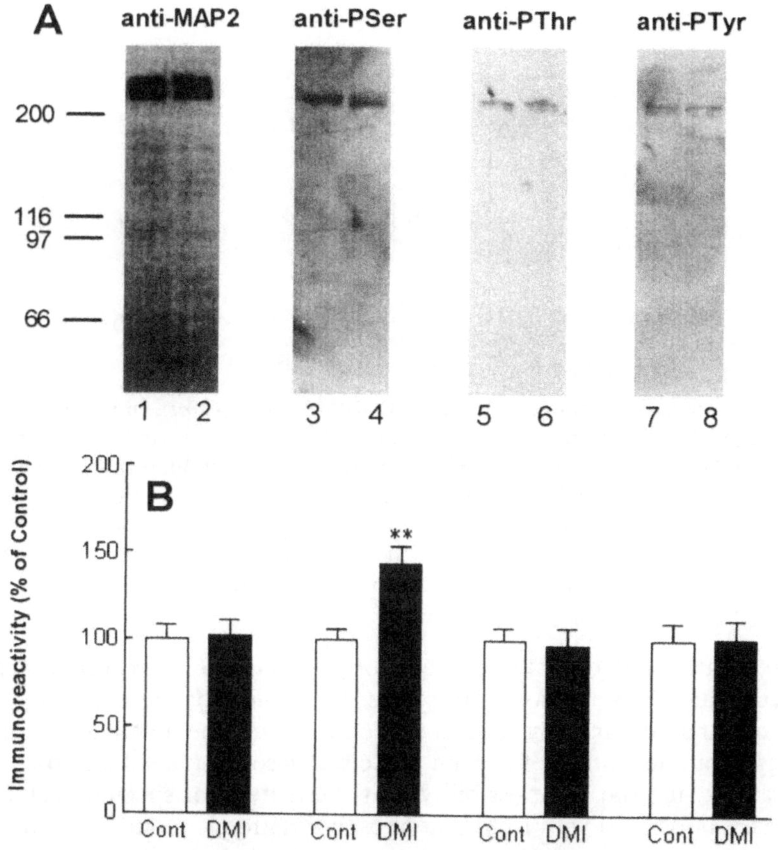

FIG. 3. (**A**) Western blot analysis of cerebrocortical boiled supernatant fraction with monoclonal antibody, *anti-MAP2* (lanes 1 and 2), antiphosphoserine (*anti-PSer*; lanes 3 and 4), antiphosphothreonine (*anti-PThr*; lanes 5 and 6), or antiphosphotyrosine (*anti-PTyr*; lanes 7 and 8) after immunoprecipitation of MAP2 from saline (lanes 1, 3, 5, 7) or desipramine-treated rats (lanes 2, 4, 6, 8) (20 mg/kg once daily for 14 days). (**B**) Histograms show the level of MAP2, phosphoserine, phosphothreonine, or phosphotyrosine immunoreactivity quantified by densitometric analysis. Each value represents the mean ± SEM of five animals in chronic saline (*Cont*) or desipramine (*DMI*) treatment group. ** $P < 0.01$: significant difference from the saline group

been reported that chronic antidepressant treatment results in a decrease in the level of PKA activity in the cytosol of the rat frontal cortex (Nestler et al. 1989). Another study has shown that chronic treatment with desipramine (10 mg/kg IP for 21 days) results in a reduction in PKC activity in both the soluble and particulate fractions of the rat cerebral cortex (Mann et al. 1995). With regard to the activity of CaM kinase II, Popoli et al. (1995) reported that long-term treatment with other antidepressants, such as fluvoxamine (a selective 5-HT reuptake inhibitor) or venlafaxine (a mixed inhibitor of 5-HT and

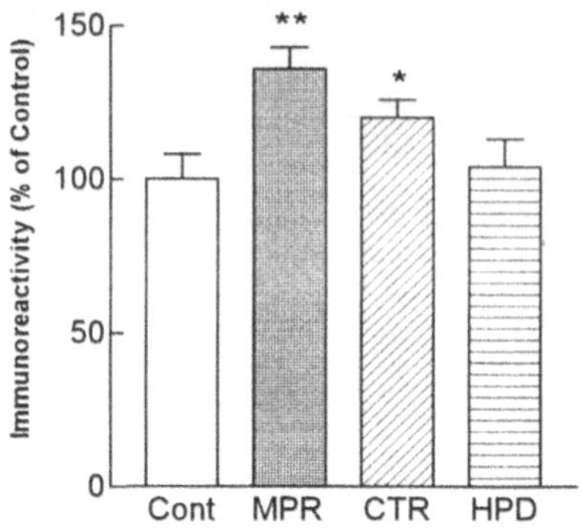

FIG. 4. Effects of long-term treatment with saline (*Cont*), maprotiline (*MPR*), citalopram (*CTR*), or haloperidol (*HPD*) for 14 days on the serine phosphorylation of MAP2 in the rat cerebrocortical boiled supernatant fraction. Immunoblotting of immunoprecipitated MAP2 with antiphosphoserine antibody was performed. Histograms show the level of phosphoserine immunoreactivity quantified by densitometric analysis. Each value represents the mean ± SEM of five animals in each treatment group. ** $P < 0.01$; * $P < 0.05$: significant difference from saline group

NE reuptake), failed to alter the level of presynaptic CaM kinase II activity in the cortical subsynaptosomal fractions. Regardless of these findings, the results of our study strongly suggest that chronic treatment with antidepressants brings about activation of certain protein kinases in the soluble fraction, but we cannot rule out the possibility that the activity of specific protein phosphatases associated with MAP2 dephosphorylation is reduced by chronic antidepressant treatment. For these reasons, further studies are necessary to determine what kinase or phosphatase could be implicated in the increased serine phosphorylation of MAP2 in response to prolonged antidepressant treatment.

Effect of Antidepressant Treatment on Microtubule Assembly

The next step of our study was to clarify the physiological role of phosphorylated MAP2 induced by chronic antidepressant treatment. Several lines of evidence demonstrate that phosphorylation of MAP2 catalyzed by several protein kinases, including type II PKA, CaM kinase II, or PKC, results in inhibition of microtubule assembly in vitro (Jameson et al. 1980; Yamamoto et al. 1985; Hoshi et al. 1988). Thus it is of interest to examine the influence of the administration of antidepressants on microtubule assembly as a possible target for the action of antidepressants. We examined microtubule assembly in the crude extracts of rat cerebral cortex in the presence or absence of a protein phosphatase inhibitor, calyculin A, to compare dephosphorylation properties

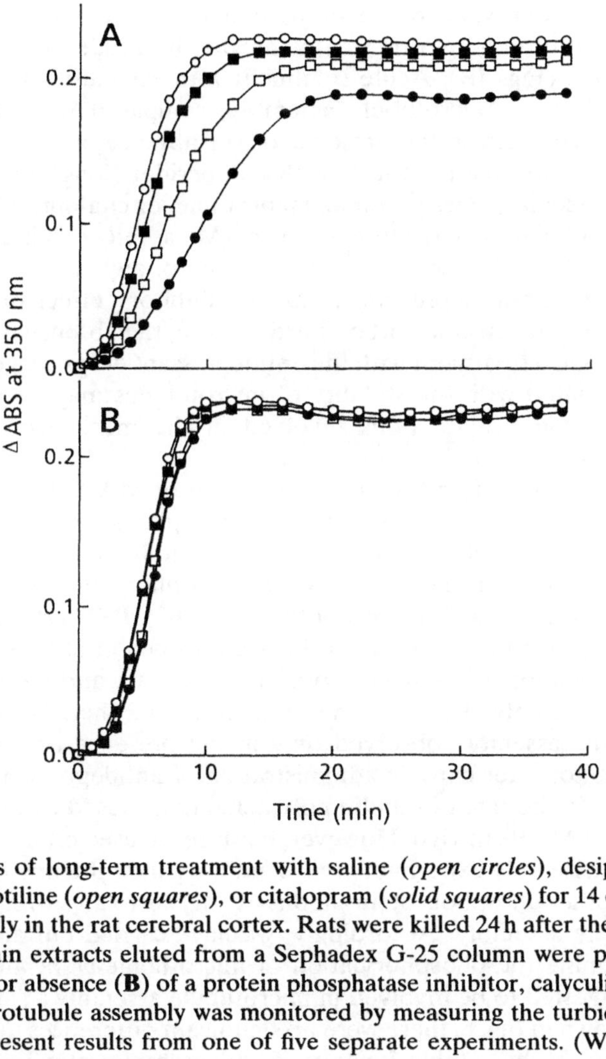

FIG. 5. Effects of long-term treatment with saline (*open circles*), desipramine (*solid circles*), maprotiline (*open squares*), or citalopram (*solid squares*) for 14 days on microtubule assembly in the rat cerebral cortex. Rats were killed 24h after the last injection. The crude brain extracts eluted from a Sephadex G-25 column were prepared in the presence (**A**) or absence (**B**) of a protein phosphatase inhibitor, calyculin A. The time course of microtubule assembly was monitored by measuring the turbidity at 350nm. The data represent results from one of five separate experiments. (With permission from Miyamoto et al., 1995a)

as described earlier (Miyamoto et al. 1995a). The assembly of tubulin into microtubules in crude brain extract in the presence of 1mM GTP was monitored by the increase in turbidity with time measured at 350nm and 37°C using a spectrophotometer.

As shown in Fig. 5A, long-term treatment with desipramine (20mg/kg SC for 14 days), maprotiline (30mg/kg), or citalopram (30mg/kg) resulted in significant decreases in the initial rate and the final extent of microtubule assembly when the buffer containing calyculin A was used to prepare the crude brain extracts. When the crude brain extracts were prepared in the absence of calyculin A, decreases in the initial rate and final extent of microtubule assembly after long-term treatment with the antidepressants were completely nullified (Fig. 5B). Acute treatment with each antidepressant had no significant effect on microtubule assembly, compared with the effects on saline-treated controls, in the presence or the absence of calyculin A. Moreover, acute and chronic treatment with haloperidol (5 mg/kg) did not affect microtubule assembly. Desipramine, maprotiline, or citalopram had no direct effect on tubulin polymerization in vitro (Miyamoto et al. 1995b). These results demonstrate that chronic administration of any of several antidepressants, but not nonantidepressants, has an inhibitory effect on microtubule assembly in the rat cerebral cortex. Furthermore, the absence of these effects in acute or in vitro treatment with the antidepressant drugs suggests that these changes associated with the stability of microtubules may be related to the long-term neuronal adaptations involved in the mechanism of action of antidepressants.

The phosphorylation and dephosphorylation of MAP2 by several protein kinases and protein phosphatases are known to play an important role in the regulation of the microtubule assembly–disassembly cycle (Yamamoto et al. 1985, 1988). It has been shown that MAP2 phosphorylated by PKA (Nishida et al. 1982), CaM kinase II (Yamamoto et al. 1985), PKC (Hoshi et al. 1988), or epidermal growth factor receptor kinase (Nishida et al. 1987) inhibits microtubule nucleation and reduces both the initial rate and the final extent of microtubule assembly in vitro (Jameson et al. 1980). Therefore the inhibition of microtubule assembly observed only in the presence of a protein phosphatase inhibitor after chronic administration of antidepressants may reflect the reduction in the rate of tubulin polymerization caused by increased phosphorylation of MAP2 in vivo. However, because we used crude extracts in the microtubule assembly experiment, we cannot exclude the possibility that the presence of other phosphoproteins in this extract correlates with the inhibition of microtubule assembly. Accordingly, we have carried out another experiment to examine the phosphorylation of microtubule-associated tau, which has been suggested to be involved in microtubule assembly (Yamamoto et al. 1985). As shown in Fig. 6, there were no significant differences in the phosphorylation of tau in the soluble fraction of the cerebral cortex between control and desipramine-treated rats. On the basis of these results, we conclude that long-term treatment of rats with antidepressants induces an increase in the degree of phosphorylation of MAP2 in vivo and has an inhibitory effect on microtubule assembly in the cerebral cortex of the rats, and that these effects may represent a novel postreceptor action of antidepressants in the intracellular signal transduction pathway.

Correlation between dendrite sprouting and an increase in MAP2 phosphorylation has been observed in cultured hippocampal neurons (Díez-Guerra and Avila 1995). It has been reported that in lamprey neurons microtubule destabilization and changes in protein phosphorylation precede dendritic sprouting (Hall et al. 1991). Nakamura (1990) has shown that repeated administration of rats with desipramine induces sprouting of noradrenergic neurons

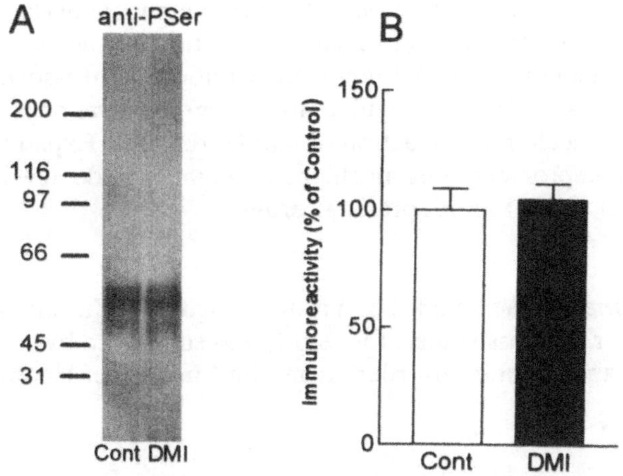

FIG. 6. Effects of long-term treatment with saline (*Cont*) or desipramine (*DMI*) for 14 days on the serine phosphorylation of tau in the rat cerebral cortex. Rats were killed 24h after the last injection. (**A**) Representative immunoblotting of immunoprecipitated tau with antiphosphoserine (*anti-PSer*) antibody. (**B**) Histograms show the level of phosphoserine immunoreactivity quantified by densitometric analysis. Each value represents the mean ± SEM of five animals in each treatment group. There are no significant differences between the two groups

in the cerebral cortex of the rats. Thus together with these findings and our results, it is conceivable that changes in MAP2 phosphorylation after chronic treatment with antidepressants can influence the stability of the microtubular network and hence induce a morphological change in dendrites.

The biochemical consequences of inhibition of microtubule assembly by chronic antidepressant treatment are unclear. It has been demonstrated that tubulin dimers, the primary constituent of microtubules, act as regulators of the adenylate cyclase signal transduction system in rat cerebral cortex membranes (Rasenick and Wang 1988; Hatta et al. 1995). These studies indicated that tubulin dimers are associated with the synaptic membrane and participate in the stimulatory or inhibitory regulation of adenylate cyclase by direct interaction as well as guanine nucleotide transfer between tubulin and G proteins. These effects are observed only for the dimer form, and not for the polymer form of tubulin. Taken together with the above results, we speculate that chronic antidepressant treatment induces an increase in the rate of formation of tubulin dimers and thus modulation of adenylate cyclase activity (Fig. 2).

Conclusion

The findings of basic studies have provided a substantial body of compelling evidence that changes in intracellular signal transduction, possibly involving protein kinases and substrate proteins, play a role in the mechanism of action of antidepressants. The regulation of the protein phosphorylation system may represent a target for antidepressants. Additional studies are required to elucidate the second messenger–phosphorylation system associated with other phosphoproteins, which may regulate long-term adaptive or plastic changes in the molecular mechanism of action of antidepressants. Expanding our knowledge of postreceptor signaling mechanisms might provide new ideas for developing novel classes of antidepressant drugs.

Acknowledgments. We thank Dr. Yasuo Sasuga, Ms. Yuriko Ogawa, and Mr. Yuji Gamo for their assistance. Our study was supported by a Research Grant for Nervous and Mental Disorders from the Ministry of Health and Welfare, Japan.

References

Akiyama T, Nishida E, Ishida J, Saji N, Ogawara H, Hoshi M, Miyata Y, Sakai H (1986) Purified protein kinase C phosphorylates microtubule-associated protein 2. J Biol Chem 261:15648–15651

Brunello N, Perez J, Tinelli D, Rovescalli AC, Racagni G (1990) Biochemical and molecular changes in rat cerebral cortex after chronic antidepressant treatment: "in vitro" and "in vivo" studies. Pharmacol Toxicol 66:112–120

Charney DS, Menkes DB, Heninger GR (1981) Receptor sensitivity and the mechanism of action of antidepressant treatment. Arch Gen Psychiatry 38:1160–1180

Díez-Guerra FJ, Avila J (1995) An increase in phosphorylation of microtubule-associated protein 2 accompanies dendrite extension during the differentiation of cultured hippocampal neurones. Eur J Biochem 227:68–77

Girault J-A (1993) Protein phosphorylation and dephosphorylation in mammalian central nervous system. Neurochem Int 23:1–25

Goldenring JR, Gonzalez B, McGuire JS Jr, DeLorenzo RJ (1983) Purification and characterization of a calmodulin-dependent kinase from rat brain cytosol able to phosphorylate tubulin and microtubule-associated proteins. J Biol Chem 258:12632–12640

Hagiwara M, Brindle P, Harootunian A, Armstrong R, Rivier J, Vale W, Tsien R, Montminy MR (1993) Coupling of hormonal stimulation and transcription via the cyclic AMP-responsive factor CREB is rate limited by nuclear entry of protein kinase A. Mol Cell Biol 13:4852–4859

Hall G, Lee VM, Kosik K (1991) Microtubule destabilization and neurofilament phosphorylation precede dendritic sprouting after close axotomy of lamprey central neurones. Proc Natl Acad Sci USA 88:5016–5020

Hatta S, Ozawa H, Saito T, Ohshika H (1995) Participation of tubulin in the stimulatory regulation of adenylyl cyclase in rat cerebral cortex membranes. J Neurochem 64:1343–1350

Hoshi M, Akiyama T, Shinohara Y, Miyata Y, Ogawara H, Nishida E, Sakai H (1988) Protein-kinase-C-catalyzed phosphorylation of the microtubule-binding domain of microtubule-associated protein 2 inhibits its ability to induce tubulin polymerization. Eur J Biochem 174:225–230

Jameson L, Frey T, Zeeberg B, Dalldorf F, Caplow M (1980) Inhibition of microtubule assembly by phosphorylation of microtubule-associated proteins. Biochemistry 19:2472–2479

Johnson GVW, Jope RS (1992) The role of microtubule-associated protein 2 (MAP-2) in neuronal growth, plasticity, and degeneration. J Neurosci Res 33:505–512

Kadowaki T, Fujita-Yamaguchi Y, Nishida E, Takaku F, Akiyama T, Kathuria S, Akanuma Y, Kasuga M (1985) Phosphorylation of tubulin and microtubule-associated proteins by the purified insulin receptor kinase. J Biol Chem 260:4016–4020

Mann CD, Vu TB, Hrdina PD (1995) Protein kinase C in rat brain cortex and hippocampus: effect of repeated administration of fluoxetine and desipramine. Br J Pharmacol 115:595–600

Melia KR, Rasmussen K, Terwilliger RZ, Haycock JW, Nestler EJ, Duman RS (1992) Coordinate regulation of the cyclic AMP system with firing rate and expression of tyrosine hydroxylase in the rat locus coeruleus: effects of chronic stress and drug treatments. J Neurochem 58:494–502

Miyamoto S, Nakanishi J, Asakura M (1993) Phosphoproteins involved in the mode of action of antidepressants and electroconvulsive shock: a possible role of cytoskeletal proteins. Jpn J Psychiatr Neurol 47:426–427

Miyamoto S, Asakura M, Sasuga Y (1995a) Effects of chronic administration of antidepressants on microtubule assembly in rat cerebral cortex. Jpn J Psychopharmacol 15:385–395

Miyamoto S, Asakura M, Sasuga Y, Imafuku J, Gamo Y, Osada K (1995b) Chronic antidepressant administration inhibits microtubule assembly in rat cerebral cortex. Eur Neuropsychopharmacol 5:280

Morinobu S, Nibuya M, Duman RS (1995) Chronic antidepressant treatment down-regulates the induction of c-fos mRNA in response to acute stress in rat frontal cortex. Neuropsychopharmacology 12:221–228

Moyer JA, Sigg EB, Silver PJ (1986) Antidepressants and protein kinases: desipramine treatment affects pineal gland cAMP-dependent protein kinase activity. Eur J Pharmacol 121:57–64

Nakamura S (1990) Antidepressants induce regeneration of catecholaminergic axon terminals in the rat cerebral cortex. Neurosci Lett 111:64–68

Nestler EJ, Walaas SI, Greengard P (1984) Neuronal phosphoproteins: physiological and clinical implications. Science 225:1357–1364

Nestler EJ, Terwilliger RZ, Duman RS (1989) Chronic antidepressant administration alters the subcellular distribution of cyclic AMP-dependent protein kinase in rat frontal cortex. J Neurochem 53:1644–1647

Nibuya M, Nestler EJ, Duman RS (1996) Chronic antidepressant administration increases the expression of cAMP response element binding protein (CREB) in rat hippocampus. J Neurosci 16:2365–2372

Nimmo HG, Cohen P (1977) Hormonal control of protein phosphorylation. Adv Cyclic Nucleotide Res 8:145–266

Nishida E, Kotani S, Kuwaki T, Sakai H (1982) Phosphorylation of microtubule-associated proteins (MAPs) controls both microtubule assembly and MAPs-actin interaction. In: Sakai H, Mohri H, Borisy GG (eds) Biological functions of microtubules and related structures. Academic, Tokyo, pp 285–295

Nishida E, Hoshi M, Miyata Y, Sakai H, Kadowaki T, Kasuga M, Saijo S, Ogawara H, Akiyama T (1987) Tyrosine phosphorylation by the epidermal growth factor receptor kinase induces functional alterations in microtubule-associated protein 2. J Biol Chem 262:16200–16204

Ozawa H, Rasenick MM (1989) Coupling of the stimulatory GTP-binding protein Gs to rat synaptic membrane adenylate cyclase is enhanced subsequent to chronic antidepressant treatment. Mol Pharmacol 36:803–808

Perez J, Tinelli D, Brunello N, Racagni G (1989) cAMP-dependent phosphorylation of soluble and crude microtubule fractions of rat cerebral cortex after prolonged desmethylimipramine treatment. Eur J Pharmacol 172:305–316

Perez J, Tinelli D, Bianchi E, Brunello N, Racagni G (1991) cAMP binding proteins in the rat cerebral cortex after administration of selective 5-HT and NE reuptake blockers with antidepressant activity. Neuropsychopharmacology 4:57–64

Peroutka SJ, Snyder SH (1980) Long-term antidepressant treatment decreases spiroperidol-labeled serotonin receptor binding. Science 210:88–90

Popoli M, Vocaturo C, Perez J, Smeraldi E, Racagni G (1995) Presynaptic Ca^{2+}/calmodulin-dependent protein kinase II: autophosphorylation and activity increase in the hippocampus after long-term blockade of serotonin reuptake. Mol Pharmacol 48:623–629

Racagni G, Brunello N, Tinelli D, Perez J (1992) New biochemical hypotheses on the mechanism of action of antidepressant drugs: cAMP-dependent phosphorylation system. Pharmacopsychiatry 25:51–55

Rasenick MM, Wang N (1988) Exchange of guanine nucleotides between tubulin and GTP-binding proteins that regulate adenylate cyclase: cytoskeletal modification of neuronal signal transduction. J Neurochem 51:300–311

Schildkraut JJ (1965) The catecholamine hypothesis of affective disorders: a review of supporting evidence. Am J Psychiatry 122:509–520

Schulman H (1984) Phosphorylation of microtubule-associated proteins by a Ca^{2+}/calmodulin-dependent protein kinase. J Cell Biol 99:11–19

Sloboda RD, Rudolph SA, Rosenbaum JL, Greengard P (1975) Cyclic AMP-dependent endogenous phosphorylation of a microtubule-associated protein. Proc Natl Acad Sci USA 72:177–181

Theurkauf WE, Vallee RB (1982) Molecular characterization of the cAMP-dependent protein kinase bound to microtubule-associated protein 2. J Biol Chem 257:3284–3290

Vallee R (1980) Structure and phosphorylation of microtubule-associated protein 2 (MAP2). Proc Natl Acad Sci USA 77:3206–3210

Vetulani J, Sulser F (1975) Action of various antidepressant treatments reduces reactivity of noradrenergic cyclic AMP-generating system in limbic forebrain. Nature 257:495–496

Walaas SI, Greengard P (1991) Protein phosphorylation and neuronal function. Pharmacol Rev 43:299–349

Walsh DA, Perkins JP, Krebs EG (1968) An adenosine 3′,5′-monophosphate-dependent protein kinase from rabbit skeletal muscle. J Biol Chem 243:3763–3774

Yamamoto H, Fukunaga K, Goto S, Tanaka E, Miyamoto E (1985) Ca^{2+},calmodulin-dependent regulation of microtubule formation via phosphorylation of microtubule-associated protein 2, τ factor, and tubulin, and comparison with the cyclic AMP-dependent phosphorylation. J Neurochem 44:759–768

Yamamoto H, Saitoh Y, Fukunaga K, Nishimura H, Miyamoto E (1988) Dephosphorylation of microtubule proteins by brain protein phosphatases 1 and 2A, and its effect on microtubule assembly. J Neurochem 50:1614–1623

Stress and BDNF Signal Transduction: Implications for Stress-Related Psychiatric Disorders

SHIGERU MORINOBU[1], MASASHI NIBUYA[2], and RONALD S. DUMAN[3]

Introduction

It is well known that stress is a major risk factor for psychiatric disorders, such as major depression and posttraumatic stress disorder (PTSD). These illnesses can have some common symptoms, such as psychogenic amnesia, diminished interest, and impaired concentration, suggesting that the underlying pathophysiology of depression and PTSD may have common features (Friedman and Yehuda 1995). Clinical studies have provided support for this possibility. Brain imaging studies have demonstrated that the volume of the hippocampus is decreased in patients with major depression (Sheline et al. 1996) or patients with PTSD (Bremner et al. 1995). These findings suggest that atrophy or death of neurons in the hippocampus may contribute to the pathogenesis of depression and PTSD. In support of this hypothesis, basic research studies have demonstrated that chronic stress causes atrophy or, in extreme cases, death of hippocampal neurons in rats and nonhuman primates.

Neurotrophic factors play a significant role not only in the development of immature neurons but also in the maintenance, function, and survival of mature neurons in the adult central nervous system (CNS). Thus it is possible that altered expression of neurotrophic factors in the CNS contributes to the atrophy and damage of hippocampal neurons. Brain-derived neurotrophic factor (BDNF) is a member of the nerve growth factor family, which also includes nerve growth factor (NGF), neurotrophin-3 (NT-3), and neurotrophin-4/5 (NT-4/5). BDNF is the most abundant neurotrophic factor in brain and is expressed throughout the CNS (Maisonpierre et al. 1990; Phillips

[1] Department of Neuropsychiatry, Yamagata University School of Medicine, 2-2-2 Iida-nishi, Yamagata 990-23, Japan
[2] Department of Psychiatry, Jichi Medical School School of Medicine, 3311-1 Yakushiji, Minamikawachi, Kawachi, Tochigi 329-04, Japan
[3] Division of Molecular Psychiatry, Department of Psychiatry, Yale University School of Medicine, 34 Park Street, New Haven, CT 06508, USA

et al. 1990). Studies have demonstrated that stress decreases the expression of BDNF in the hippocampus, suggesting that down-regulation of this neurotrophic factor could mediate, in part, the stress-induced atrophy of hippocampal neurons (Smith et al. 1995). Moreover, it is possible that the up-regulation of BDNF expression may prevent the atrophy and damage of hippocampal neurons in response to stress.

Physiological Functions of BDNF

Several neurotrophic functions specific to BDNF are shown in Table 1. BDNF is reported to support the differentiation and survival of neurons. For instance, Hyman and her co-workers (1994) demonstrated that BDNF, as well as NT-3, promotes the survival and differentiation of dopaminergic neurons in the rat brain. Mamounas and her colleagues (1995) demonstrated that local infusion of BDNF into rat frontoparietal cortex prevents the severe loss of serotonin (5-hydroxytryptamine, 5-HT) axons in response to treatment with the neurotoxin *p*-chloroamphetamine (PCA) and enhances the survival and sprouting of damaged 5-HT axons. Moreover, BDNF is reported to activate dopamine and 5-HT metabolism and potentiate behaviors related to these neurotransmitter systems (Martin-Iverson et al. 1994). For example, local infusion of BDNF into the midbrain is reported to have antidepressant effects in rat behavioral models of depression, including the forced swim and learned helplessness paradigms (Siuciak et al. 1994). These findings demonstrate that BDNF has neuroprotective effects and suggest that this neurotrophic factor may have therapeutic value for the treatment of neurodegenerative diseases and psychiatric illnesses, including depression and PTSD.

Regulation of BDNF Expression

The activation of several types of neurotransmitter receptor has been shown to modulate the expression of BDNF in cultured cells and in rat brain. For example, stimulation of non-NMDA receptors by kainic acid strikingly en-

TABLE 1. Physiological functions of BDNF

Acetylcholine: supports the survival and differentiation of cholinergic neurons in the basal forebrain
Dopamine: promotes the survival and differentiation of dopaminergic neurons
Serotonin: prevents the severe loss of axons and enhances the survival of damaged axons caused by *p*-chloroamphetamine in frontoparietal cortex

BDNF, brain-derived neurotrophic factor.

hances BDNF mRNA levels in primary cultures of hippocampal neurons and intact rat hippocampus (Zafra et al. 1990); and inhibition of GABA receptors by bicuculline significantly increases BDNF mRNA levels in rat hippocampus (Zafra et al. 1991). In addition, the stimulation of muscarinic receptors by pilocarpine markedly increases BDNF mRNA levels in both early postnatal and adult rat hippocampus (Berzaghi et al. 1993). Monoamine neurotransmitters, including norepinephrine and dopamine, are reported to significantly enhance BDNF mRNA in primary cultures of astrocytes (Zafra et al. 1992).

Although the intracellular signal transduction pathways that control the expression of BDNF mRNA have not been completely characterized, activation of the cAMP system is reported to increase the expression of BDNF. Treatment of cultured cells with forskolin, an activator of adenylate cyclase, increases the expression of BDNF mRNA (Zafra et al. 1992). Moreover, treatment of primary astroglial cultures with the phosphodiesterase inhibitor 3-isobutyl-1-methylxanthine (IBMX) is reported to increase levels of BDNF expression (Condorelli et al. 1994). These results suggest that activation of receptors coupled to the cAMP system, such as the β_1-adrenoceptor and 5-HT-4, 5-HT-6, and 5-HT-7 receptors, may increase the expression of BDNF (Fig. 1). Regulation of neuronal gene expression by the cAMP system is mediated by cAMP-dependent protein kinases and the cAMP response element binding protein (CREB), a major transcription factor by this second messenger system. CREB regulates gene transcription via binding to cAMP response element (CRE) sites located in the promoter regions of genes. Interestingly, CREB can also be phosphorylated and activated by calcium-dependent kinases (i.e., calcium/calmodulin-dependent protein kinase and protein kinase C). In this way, CREB may act as a common intracellular target of receptors coupled to the calcium-dependent kinases, such as 5-HT-2 and α_1-adrenergic receptors. It is also possible that CREB acts as a common target for antidepressant drugs that have their acute effects via activation of monoamine receptors coupled to either cAMP or calcium-regulated pathways.

BDNF Signal Transduction Cascade

The exact mechanisms by which BDNF and other neurotrophic factors influence the differentiation and survival of neurons in the CNS is still unknown. Studies have revealed that the protein tyrosine kinase TrkB is a component of a high-affinity receptor for BDNF (Glass and Yancopoulos 1993). The Trk receptors contain an extracellular binding domain and an intracellular tyrosine kinase domain. A possible intracellular signal transduction cascade for activated TrkB is shown in Fig. 2. The binding of BDNF to TrkB receptor results in autophosphorylation of tyrosine residues on the intracellular domain of the receptor. Subsequently, intracellular poteins that contain SH2 domains can

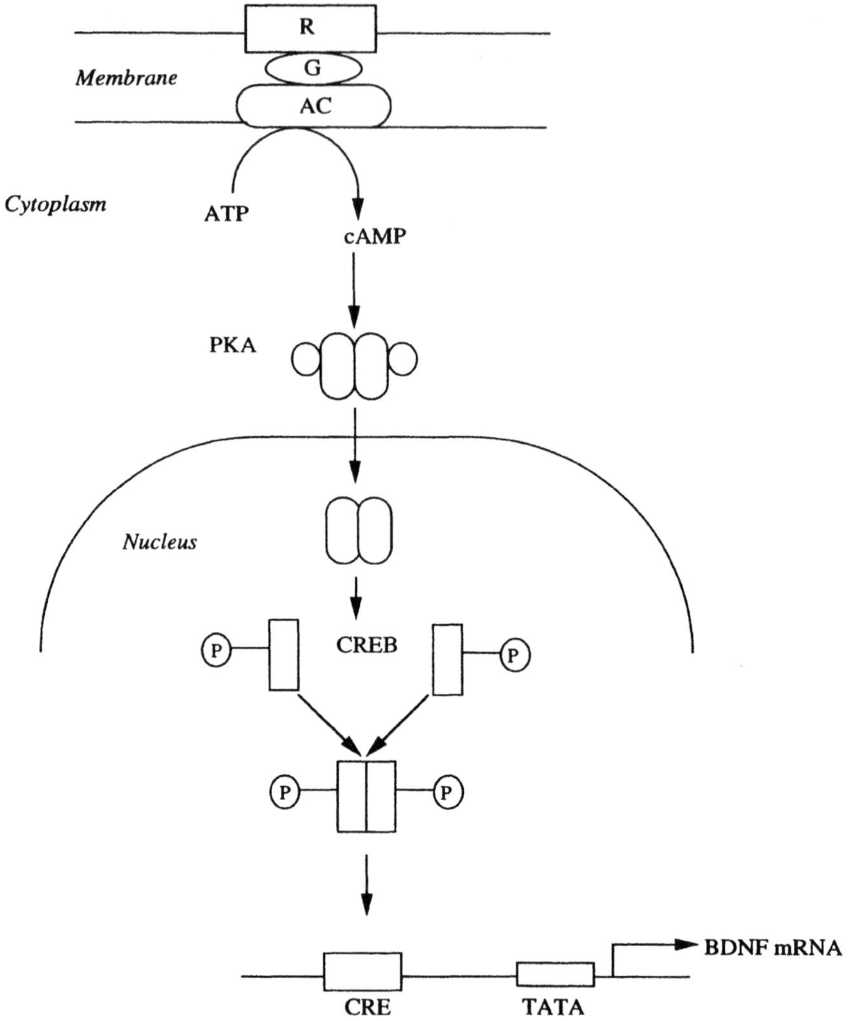

FIG. 1. Regulation of brain-derived neurotrophic factor (BDNF) mRNA expression mediated by the cyclic adenosine monophosphate (cAMP) system. *PKA*, protein kinase A; *R*, receptor; *G*, G protein; *AC*, adenylate cyclase; *CREB*, cAMP response element binding protein; *CRE*, cAMP response element; *P*, phosphorylation

interact with intracellular domains of the TrkB receptor. This interaction may induce the activation of Ras and a protein kinase cascade including mitogen-activated protein (MAP) kinase. Activation of the MAP kinase pathway is reported to have multiple functions, including regulation of specific gene transcription factors. In this context, it is thought that BDNF exerts its physiological function in the CNS via the TrkB–MAP kinase pathway.

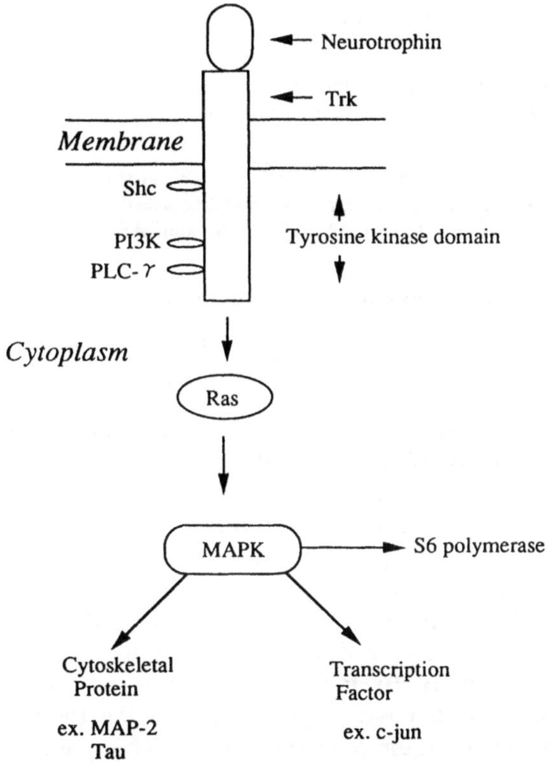

FIG. 2. Signal transduction pathway through the neurotrophin receptor *Trk*. *Shc*, Shc protein; *PI3K*, phosphatidylinositol-3 kinase; *PLC-γ*, phospholipase C-γ; *MAPK*, mitogenactivated protein; *MAP2*, microtuble associated protein 2

Stress-Induced Hippocampal Cellular Damage

Several studies have demonstrated that chronic stress produces atrophy and damage of neurons in the hippocampus (Table 2). Chronic restraint stress or glucocorticoid treatments are reported to cause atrophy of the apical dendrites of CA3 pyramidal neurons in rat hippocampus (Watanabe et al. 1992). This atrophy is expressed as a decrease in the number and length of dendritic branch points of CA3 pyramidal neurons. In addition, exposure to prolonged stress is reported to cause marked neuronal degeneration of hippocampal neurons of vervet monkeys (Uno et al. 1989). That study reported that the pyramidal neurons throughout the CA regions are shrunken and sparse, and that several ultrastructural changes, such as the loss of Nissl bodies or decrease in perikaryon size, are observed in hippocampal CA3, CA1, and CA4 pyramidal neurons. This evidence suggests that chronic stress and hypersecretion of

TABLE 2. Hippocampal damage associated with chronic stress

Rat	
	Decrease in the number and length of dendritic branch points of CA3 pyramidal neurons
	Atrophy of apical dendrites of CA3 pyramidal neurons
Monkey	
	Shrunken and sparse pyramidal neurons throughout the CA regions
	Loss of Nissl bodies in CA3, CA1, and CA4 pyramidal neurons
	Decrease in perikaryon size in CA3, CA1, and CA4 pyramidal neurons
Human	
	Hippocampal atrophy in patients with posttraumatic stress disorder or recurrent major depression

glucocorticoids may induce neuronal degeneration in the hippocampus (Sapolsky et al. 1990; Wooley et al. 1990).

Neuroimaging studies have revealed that there are morphological alterations in the brains with major depression or PTSD. The results demonstrate that the volume of hippocampus is decreased with these psychiatric disorders. Sheline and colleagues (1996) used magnetic resonance imaging (MRI) to examine the size of the hippocampus in depressed patients. They found that there are decreases of 12% and 15% in the volumes of the right and left hippocampus, respectively. Bremner and co-workers (1995), also using MRI, found that PTSD patients have a significantly smaller right hippocampal volume relative to that of their control subjects. The results of these clinical studies support the hypothesis that stress causes atrophy and damage to hippocampal neurons and raises the possibility that these effects may be closely associated with the pathogenesis of major depression and PTSD. Thus it is important to elucidate the mechanisms by which stress and glucocorticoid treatments cause neuronal degeneration of the hippocampus. It is conceivable that progress in this area may lead to new pharmacotherapeutic strategies for the treatment of stress-related psychiatric illnesses.

Stress and BDNF

Given the importance of BDNF and other neurotrophic factors in the survival and function of neurons, it is possible that decreased expression of neurotrophic factors could contribute to the stress-induced atrophy of hippocampal neurons. Smith and colleagues (1995) reported that both acute and chronic restraint stress significantly decrease BDNF mRNA levels in the CA3 pyramidal and dentate gyrus granule cell layers of hippocampus. In addition, the reduction of BDNF mRNA is mediated, at least in part, by elevated levels of corticosterone in rats (Smith et al. 1995). Nibuya and colleagues (1995) replicated the effects of acute stress on expression of BDNF mRNA and demonstrated that chronic administration of antidepressants prevents the reduction of BDNF mRNA in response to acute stress in rat hippocampus. We have also

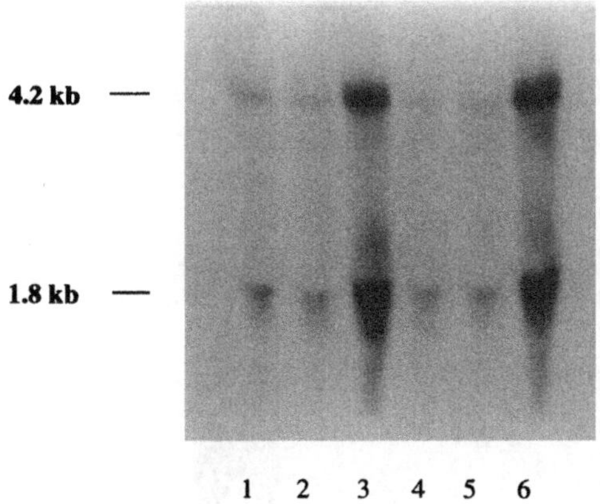

FIG. 3. Northern blot analysis of BDNF mRNA in hippocampus of rats subjected to acute stress and posttreatment with various antidepressants. *1*, handling + saline; *2*, stress + saline; *3*, stress + ECS (electroconvulsive seizure); *4*, stress + imipramine; *5*, stress + tranylcypromine; *6*, stress + ECS

investigated the influence of acute antidepressant treatments on the stress-induced down-regulation of BDNF mRNA in hippocampus. Acute posttreatment with electroconvulsive seizure (ECS), but not imipramine or tranylcypromine, significantly increased BDNF mRNA levels (Figs. 3, 4). These results indicate that blockade of the stress-induced down-regulation of BDNF is dependent on chronic administration of antidepressant drugs, but that this effect is immediately reversed by acute ECS. Moreover, the results suggest that up-regulation of BDNF may contribute to the therapeutic actions of antidepressant treatments. This possibility is supported by the behavioral studies, cited above, demonstrating that BDNF has antidepressant effects in animal models of depression (Siuciak et al. 1994).

Co-Administration of a Phosphodiesterase Inhibitor and the Response to Selective Norepinephrine Reuptake Inhibitor

Levels of BDNF mRNA in rat hippocampus are reported to be significantly increased by acute and chronic administration of ECS or several types of antidepressant (Nibuya et al. 1995). In addition, chronic ECS or antidepressants significantly increase the expression and function of CREB in rat hippocampus (Nibuya et al. 1996). Previous studies have demonstrated that chronic administration of antidepressants regulates the density of β-adrenergic receptor binding and levels of mRNA (Hosoda and Duman, 1993). In addition, antidepressant treatments are reported to increase levels of cAMP-dependent protein kinase and to cause translocation of this kinase to crude nuclear

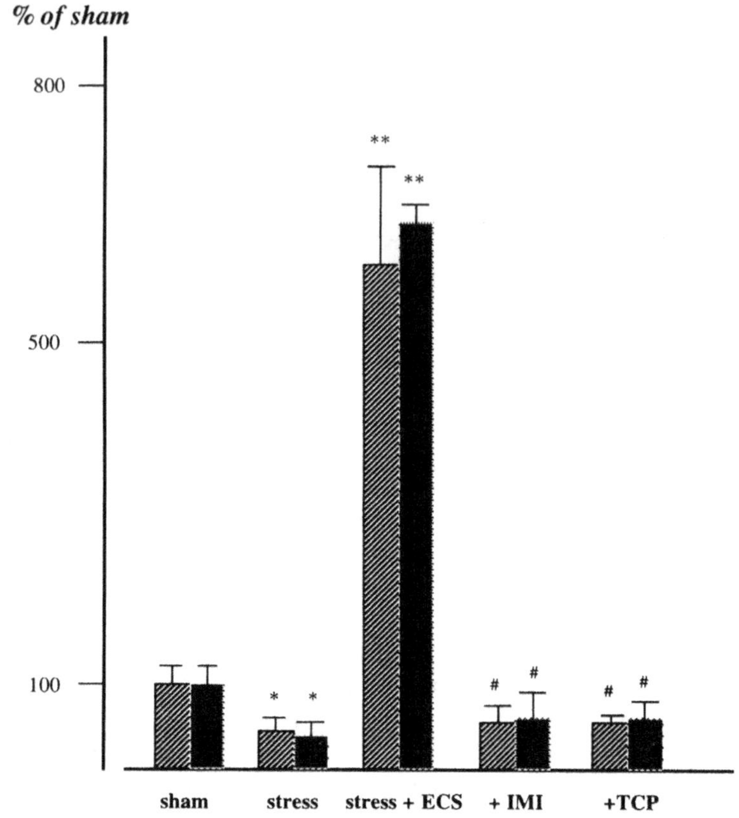

FIG. 4. Influence of acute stress and posttreatment with various types of antidepressants on BDNF mRNA expression in rat hippocampus. The results are expressed as percent of sham (100%) and are the mean ± SEM of three to six rats for each treatment group. Upper band (*hatched bars*) indicates the 4.2-kb band, and lower band (*dotted bars*) indicates the 1.8-kb band. The indicated groups are found to be significantly different from the saline-treated group (ANOVA with Fisher's test). $*P < 0.05$; $**P < 0.01$; $^{\#}P < 0.1$. *Sham*, handling + saline; *Stress*, stress + saline; *+IMI*, stress + imipramine; *+TCP*, stress + tranylcypromine

fractions of cerebral cortex (Nestler et al. 1989). These fingings indicate that antidepressant treatments activate the cAMP signal transduction cascade and suggest that antidepressant regulation of BDNF mRNA is mediated by this second messenger system.

Based on these findings, it is possible that enhancement of cAMP levels increases or potentiates the expression of BDNF mRNA. A possible way to increase cellular levels of cAMP is with the use of phosphodiesterase (PDE) inhibitors, agents that block the breakdown of cAMP. Nibuya and colleagues (1996) reported that chronic administration of PDE inhibitors increases the

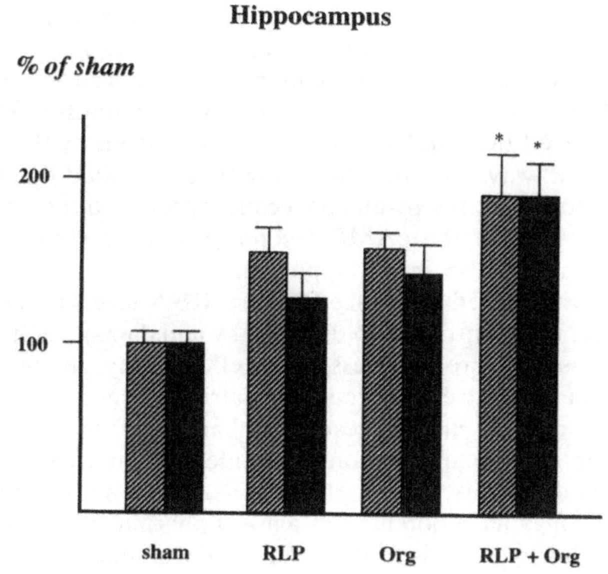

FIG. 5. Influence of chronic vehicle, rolipram (*RLP*), Org 4428 (*Org*), and rolipram plus Org 4428 (*RLP + Org*) on levels of BDNF mRNA in rat hippocampus. The results are expressed as percent of sham (vehicle-treated group) (100%) and are the mean ± SEM of six rats for each treatment group. The groups are found to be significantly different from the saline-treated group (ANOVA with Fisher's test). $*P < 0.05$. *Hatched bars*, upper band (4.2 kb); *dotted bars*, lower band (1.8 kb)

expression of BDNF, as well as CREB, in rat hippocampus. In addition, co-administration of a PDE inhibitor was found to enhance the induction of BDNF mRNA in response to tricyclic antidepressants. We have investigated the influence of acute or chronic co-administration of rolipram, a selective PDE type IV inhibitor, with Org 4428, a selective norepinephrine reuptake inhibitor (SNRI), on the expression of BDNF mRNA in rat hippocampus. Levels of BDNF mRNA were determined after acute (2 h after a single treatment) or chronic (2 h after the last treatment, for 21 days) co-administration of rolipram (1.25 mg/kg IP) with Org 4428 (20 mg/kg IP). Northern blot analysis demonstrates that whereas acute co-administration does not change levels of BDNF mRNA, chronic co-administration of rolipram markedly enhances the induction of BDNF mRNA levels by Org 4428 in rat hippocampus (Fig. 5).

Conclusion

Clinical studies of depression indicate that the repeated, chronic administration of antidepressants is required for effective treatment. This evidence suggests that the therapeutic action of antidepressants may be induced by long-term adaptations of neuronal function. Such adaptations may occur via regulation of neurotransmitter receptors, second messengers, and transcription factors, even though the acute pharmacological action of antidepressants is inhibition of monoamine reuptake or metabolism. Several studies have demonstrated that BDNF expression is regulated by the cAMP signal transduction pathway, and that this pathway is regulated by antidepressant treatments. Moreover, the results of recent reports and the present study indicate that activation of the cAMP second messenger system leads to enhanced expression of BDNF in rat hippocampus.

Stress is reported to reduce BDNF mRNA levels in the hippocampus, and this effect may contribute to the atrophy and damage of hippocampal neurons in response to chronic stress. Such effects may, in turn, contribute to the pathogenesis of stress-related psychiatric disorders, such as depression and PTSD. The results also suggest that enhancement of BDNF expression may be a relevant therapeutic action of antidepressant treatments. In this regard, recent findings raise the possibility that co-administration of rolipram with Org 4428 may have potential as a novel pharmacotherapy for depression and PTSD. This hypothesis requires additional studies to examine the efficacy of the co-administration strategy and to examine the potential side effects of rolipram.

References

Berzaghi MP, Cooper J, Castrén E, Zafra F, Sofroniew M, Thoenen H, Lindholm D (1993) Cholinergic regulation of brain-derived neurotrophic factor (BDNF) but not neurotrophin-3 (NT-3) mRNA levels in the developing rat hippocampus. J Neurosci 13:3818–3826

Bremner JD, Randall P, Scott T, Bronen RA, Seibyl JP, Southwick SM, Delaney RC, McCarthy G, Charney DS, Innis RB (1995) MRI-based measurement of hippocampal volume in patients with combat-related posttraumatic stress disorder. Am J Psychiatry 152:973–981

Condorelli DF, Dell'Albani PD, MudòG, Timmusk T, Belluardo N (1994) Expression of neurotrophins and their receptors in primary astroglial culture: induction by cyclic AMP-elevating agents. J Neurochem 63:509–516

Friedman MJ, Yehuda R (1995) Post-traumatic stress disorder and comorbidity. In: Friedman MJ, Charney DS, Deutch AY (eds) Neurobiology and clinical consequences of stress. Lippincott-Raven, Philadelphia, pp 429–445

Glass DJ, Yancopoulos GD (1993) The neurotrophins and their receptors. Trends Cell Biol 3:262–268

Hosoda K, Duman RS (1993) Regulation of β-adrenergic receptor mRNA and ligand binding by antidepressant treatments and norepinephrine depletion in rat frontal cortex. J Neurochem 60:1335–1343

Hyman C, Juhasz M, Jackson C, Wright P, Ip NY, Lindsay RM (1994) Overlapping and distinct actions of the neurotrophins BDNF, NT-3, and NT-4/5 on cultured dopaminergic and GABAergic neurons of the ventral mesencephalon. J Neurosci 14:335–347

Maisonpierre PC, Belluscio L, Squinto S, Ip NY, Furth ME, Lindsay RM, Yancopoulos GD (1990) Neurotrophin-3: a neurotrophic factor related to NGF and BDNF. Science 247:1446–1451

Mamounas LA, Blue ME, Siuciak JA, Altar CA (1995) Brain-derived neurotrophic factor promotes the survival and sprouting of serotonergic axons in rat brain. J Neurosci 15:7929–7939

Martin-Iverson MT, Todd KG, Altar CA (1994) Brain-derived neurotrophic factor and neurotrophin-3 activate striatal dopamine and serotonin metabolism and related behaviors: interactions with amphetamine. J Neurosci 14:1262–1270

Nestler RJ, Terwilliger RZ, Duman RS (1989) Chronic antidepressant administration alters the subcellular distribution of cyclic AMP-dependent protein kinase in rat frontal cortex. J Neurochem 53:1644–1647

Nibuya M, Morinobu S, Duman RS (1995) Regulation of BDNF and TrkB mRNA in rat brain by chronic electroconvulsive seizure and antidepressant drug treatments. J Neurosci 15:7539–7547

Nibuya M, Nestler EJ, Duman RS (1996) Chronic antidepressant administration increases the expression of cAMP response element binding protein (CREB) in rat hippocampus. J Neurosci 16:2365–2372

Phillips HS, Heins JM, Winslow JW (1990) Widespread expression of BDNF but not NT-3 by target areas of basal forebrain cholinergic neurons. Science 250:2914–2919

Sapolsky RM, Uno H, Robert CS, Finsh CE (1990) Hippocampal damage associated with prolonged glucocorticoid exposure in primates. J Neurosci 10:2897–2902

Sheline YI, Wang PW, Gado MH, Csernansky JG, Vannier MW (1996) Hippocampal atrophy in recurrent major depression. Proc Natl Sci USA 93:3908–3913

Siuciak JA, Lewis D, Wiegand SJ, Lindsay RM (1994) Brain derived neurotrophic factor (BDNF) produces an anti-depressant like effect in two animal models of depression. Soc Neurosci Abstr 20:1106

Smith MA, Makino S, Kvetnansky R, Post RM (1995) Stress and glucocorticoids affect the expression of brain-derived neurotrophic factor and neurotrophin-3 mRNAs in the hippocampus. J Neurosci 15:1768–1777

Uno H, Tarara R, Else JG, Suleman MA, Sapolsky RM (1989) Hippocampal damage associated with prolonged and fatal stress in primates. J Neurosci 9:1705–1711

Watanabe Y, Gould E, McEwen BS (1992) Stress induces atrophy of apical dendrites of hippocampal CA3 pyramidal neurons. Brain Res 588:341–345

Wooley CS, Gould E, McEwen BS (1990) Exposure to excess glucocorticoid alters dendritic morphology of adult hippocampal pyramidal neurons. Brain Res 588:341–345

Zafra F, Hengerer B, Thoenen H, Lindholm D (1990) Activity dependent regulation of BDNF and NGF mRNAs in the rat hippocampus is mediated by non-NMDA glutamate receptors. EMBO 11:3545–3550

Zafra F, Castrén E, Thoenen H, Lindholm D (1991) Interplay between glutamate and γ-aminobutyric acid transmitter systems in the physiological regulation of brain-derived neurotrophic factor and nerve growth factor synthesis in hippocampal neurons. Proc Natl Acad Sci USA 88:10037–10041

Zafra F, Lindholm D, Castrén E, Hartikka J, Thoenen H (1992) Regulation of brain-derived neurotrophic factor and nerve growth factor mRNA in primary cultures of hippocampal neurons and astrocytes. J Neurosci 12:4793–4799

Postreceptor Signal-Transduction Systems as Potential Targets of Lithium

Y. ODAGAKI, N. NISHI, and T. KOYAMA

Introduction

All cells have the capacity to receive external information and to transduce it to intracellular signals ending in physiological responses specific to the cell type. The rapid advance in neuroscience has elucidated the molecular mechanisms underlying such transmembrane signaling pathways. The extracellular information transmitted by hormones, neurotransmitters, and neuromodulators is recognized by specific protein molecules at the cell surface (receptors), which constitute ion channels themselves or modulate intracellular enzymatic machinery, resulting in alteration of second-messenger levels via guanine nucleotide-binding regulatory (G) proteins. The former type of receptor, the ligand-gated ion channels, also known as ionotropic receptors, includes nicotinic acetylcholine, serotonin$_3$ (5-HT$_3$), γ-aminobutyric acid$_A$ (GABA$_A$), and excitatory amino acid receptors, such as *N*-methyl-D-aspantate (NMDA), α-amino-3-hydroxy-5-methylisoxazole-4-propionate (AMPA), and kinate subtypes, that respond to the agonist-induced stimulation within milliseconds. The latter type of receptor, the G-protein-coupled or metabotropic receptors, includes adrenergic, serotonergic (except for 5-HT$_3$ receptors), dopaminergic, muscarinic acetylcholine, opioid, adenosine, GABA$_B$, metabotropic glutamate, and many neuropeptide receptors. This type of receptor couples with second-messenger-generating enzymes, such as adenylyl cyclase, phospholipase C, cyclic guanosine monophosphate (GMP) phosphodiesterase, and phospholipase A$_2$, as well as several ion channels, through the respective G proteins, thus mediating much slower signaling than the ionotropic receptors. Signal-transduction systems mediated through G-protein-coupled receptors are of great interest to biological psychiatrists, since the substances that have been supposed to be involved in the mechanisms of action of psychotropic drugs as well as in the pathophysiology of various

Department of Psychiatry, Hokkaido University School of Medicine, North 15, West 7, Kita-ku, Sapporo, Hokkaido 060, Japan psychiatric illnesses for the last few decades, such as noradrenaline, dopamine, and 5-HT, interact almost exclusively with this type of receptor.

Conventionally, receptor subtypes have been defined by their pharmacological characteristics determined by using selective agonists and antagonists. The rapid development of molecular biological techniques has nowadays made it possible to differentiate receptor subtypes structurally, even if selective agonists or antagonists are not available, and sometimes even when their functional roles and coupled second-messenger-generating systems are unknown. The number of identified receptor subtypes is still expanding.

G-protein-mediated signal transduction across the cell membrane has been summarized as follows (Gilman 1987; Birnbaumer et al. 1990). When the receptor is activated by an agonist, its conformation is altered so that the receptor interacts with heterotrimeric G proteins composed of α, β, and γ subunits. Subsequently, the α subunit of the G protein is conformationally changed to release guanosine diphosphate (GDP) from its guanine nucleotide-binding site, which is displaced by GTP. The GTP-bound, active form of the α subunit (α_{GTP}) is dissociated from βγ subunits and regulates the activity of the effector enzyme to alter the concentration of second messenger. The activated phase of the G protein is terminated by the hydrolysis of GTP bound to the α subunit catalyzed by a GTPase enzyme intrinsic to the α subunit. The GDP-bound, inactive α subunit (α_{GDP}) is then reassociated with βγ subunits to end the activation cycle. In general, it has been assumed that the specificity of the G protein for the receptor subtype as well as for the effector depends on the α subunit (Spiegel et al. 1992). Recently, however, the role of βγ subunits has also been emphasized (Birnbaumer 1992; Iñiguez-Lluhi et al. 1993).

The nomenclature of G proteins was originally based on their functional characteristics. The G proteins involved in the regulation of adenylyl cyclase activity were designated G_s and G_i, depending on their stimulatory or inhibitory mode of regulation, respectively. The other G protein, which was purified from brain with its definite function unknown, was then named G_o. Although this pharmacological classification of G proteins is still of importance as a frame of reference, a growing body of G-protein subtypes have been identified and designated by molecular cloning, not only for the α subunit but also for the β and γ subunits, as in the case of receptor subclassification (Hepler and Gilman 1992). The heterogeneity of the component proteins, together with the complexity of the network of synaptic connections as well as possible cross-talk between separate signaling pathways in the same cell, permits a delicate and dynamic tuning of neuronal activity, with divergence in some cases and convergence in other cases of multiple signaling (Gudermann et al. 1997), resulting in harmonious higher brain function and fine-tuned homeostasis in a living organism.

Previously, almost all research on the mode of action of psychotropic agents was concerned with presynaptic events or, at most, cell-surface receptors of a certain single neurotransmitter signaling system. In the case of lithium, especially, despite numerous studies in relation to 5-HT, dopamine, noradrenaline, acetylcholine, and GABA neurotransmission (Lenox and Manji 1995), the mechanism of action of this mood-stabilizing drug is still unclear. In the last several years, with the expanding knowledge of receptor-mediated intracellular signal-transduction systems, many researchers have directed their attention to postreceptor signal-transduction pathways as potential targets of the therapeutic action of this monovalent ion. This chapter reviews the reports on the effects of lithium, focusing on the components of postreceptor signal-transduction systems mediated by G-protein-coupled receptors.

Lithium and Postreceptor Signal-Transduction

Phosphoinositide Metabolism

The main pathways of phosphatidylinositol metabolism and postulated sites of action of lithium are shown in Fig. 1. To conceptualize the complicated recycling systems of phosphoinositides, the reader is referred to the extensive and excellent review by Rana and Hokin (1990). In addition, several reviews focusing on the relevance of this second-messenger system to the therapeutic action of lithium are helpful (Drummond 1987; Baraban et al. 1989; Berridge et al. 1989; Nahorski et al. 1991).

The first epoch-making finding in this field was reported by Allison and Stewart (1971), who showed that the brain inositol concentration was decreased after the injection of lithium. This finding was confirmed repeatedly by the same group and other investigators, and the concomitant increase in inositol monophosphate (IP_1) concentration after lithium administration was demonstrated in those reports (Allison et al. 1976; Sherman et al. 1981, 1985, 1986; Hirvonen and Savolainen, 1991). These phenomena in vivo, that is, decrease in inositol and increase in IP_1 concentration after lithium administration, have been attributed to the in vitro inhibitory effect of lithium on inositol monophosphatase, a key enzyme that catalyzes the dephosphorylation of IP_1 to free inositol (Hallcher and Sherman 1980; Sherman et al. 1981; Takimoto et al. 1985; Ackermann et al. 1987; Attwood et al. 1988; Gee et al. 1988a). The most noticeable point of these studies is that lithium inhibits inositol monophosphatase, with concentrations of around 1 m*M* causing 50% inhibition, since these concentrations are within its narrow therapeutically effective range in clinical practice. Another important finding is that lithium inhibits the enzyme in an uncompetitive manner. This mode of inhibitory action of lithium indicates that lithium exerts its efficacy more prominently when the phosphoinositide turnover is overactivated by excessive stimuli, which suitably explains the characteristics of lithium as an antimanic drug in clinical situations (Nahorski et al. 1991). On the basis of these results, Berridge et al. (1982) used lithium to provide an in vitro method for measuring agonist-induced phosphoinositide-hydrolyzing activity, by means of which subsequent investigations on the receptors associated with phosphoinositide turnover were greatly facilitated. In addition, they proposed a hypothesis that lithium exerts its therapeutic action by inhibiting inositol monophosphatase, leading to a lower inositol level and thus reduced receptor-coupled phosphoinositide

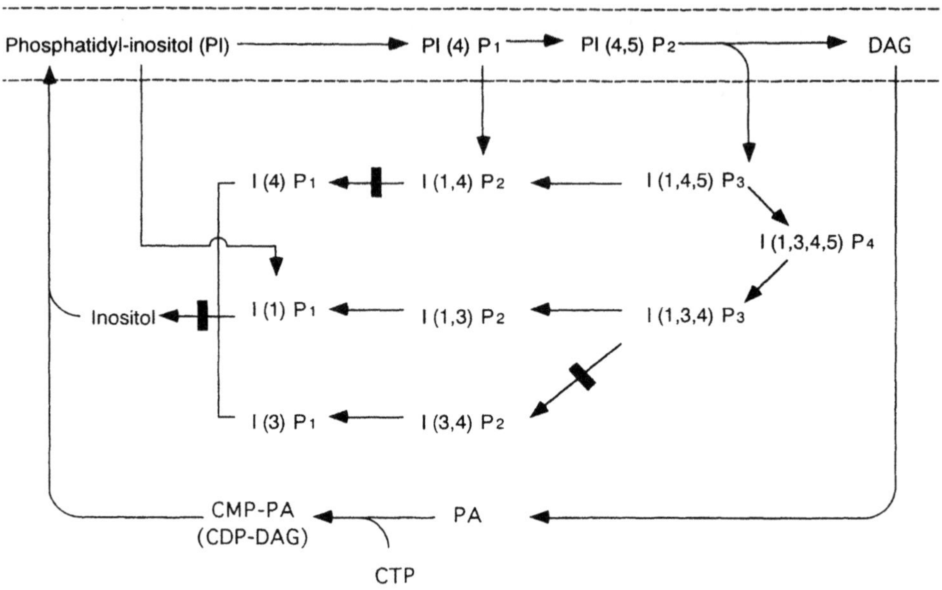

FIG. 1. The phosphoinositide cycle in mammalian cells and its sensitivity to blockade by lithium. Agonist-dependent hydrolysis of phosphatidylinositol 4,5-bisphosphate [*PI(4,5)P₂*] by phospholipase C generates two second messengers: inositol 1,4,5-trisphosphate [*I(1,4,5)P₃*], which facilitates the release of intracellular stored Ca^{2+}, and sn-2-diacylglycerol (*DAG*), which activates PKC. I(1,4,5)P_3 is phosphorylated by a 3-kinase to the putative second messenger inositol 1,3,4,5-tetrakisphosphate [*I(1,3,4,5)*P_4] or dephosphorylated by a 5-phosphatase to inositol 1,4-bisphosphate [*I(1,4)*P_2]. The indicated dephosphorylation pathways by the two enzymes are shown to be inhibited by lithium in a noncompetitive manner: inositol polyphosphate 1-phosphatase, which dephosphorylates inositol 1,3,4-trisphosphate [*I(1,3,4)*P_3] and I(1,4)P_2, and inositol monophosphatase, which dephosphorylates all of the inositol monophosphate isomers [*I(4)*P_1, *I(1)*P_1, *and I(3)*P_1]. DAG is metabolized via phosphatidic acid (PA) and cytidine monophosphate-phosphatidate (*CMP-PA*) also referred to as CDP-diacylglycerol (*CPD-DAG*) and, in conjunction with free inositol, is used to resynthesize phosphatidylinositol

hydrolysis, especially in those neurons that are being stimulated excessively (Berridge et al. 1982). This inositol-depletion hypothesis is persuasive when the special situation of the brain is considered. Because the neuronal cells in the central nervous system are unable to take up plasma inositol and are dependent on the de novo synthesis of inositol from glucose, the inhibition by lithium of the conversion to inositol of an inositol monophosphate intermediate [I(3)P_1] synthesized from glucose leads to selective deterioration of phosphoinositide turnover in the central nervous system (Drummond 1987). In addition to its inhibitory effect on inositol monophosphatase, lithium has been shown to inhibit uncompetitively another enzyme, inositol polyphosphate 1-phosphatase, as indicated in Fig. 1 (Inhorn and Majerus 1987; Gee et al. 1988b). These multiple sites of action of lithium in vitro should be taken into consideration when interpreting time-dependent and varied, sometimes inconsistent, results concerning the further detailed effects of lithium on the individual components of the phosphoinositide-hydrolyzing system under different experimental conditions (Batty and Nahorski 1985, 1987; Sherman et al. 1985; Ackermann et al. 1987; Whitworth and Kendall 1988; Kennedy et al. 1989; Kendall and Whitworth 1990; Dixon et al. 1992; Jope et al. 1992; Lee et al. 1992). Furthermore, in experiments with brain slices in vitro, the depletion of inositol resulting from the experimental conditions must have a substantial influence upon the effects of lithium on phosphoinositide turnover, which may complicate the interpretation of the data (Stubbs and Agranoff 1993). Indeed, several investigations have shown that lithium-induced alterations in some indexes of phosphoinositide hydrolysis are antagonized by the addition of inositol (Whitworth and Kendall 1988; Kennedy et al. 1989, 1990; Godfrey 1989; Brami et al. 1993; Heacock et al. 1993). The extent of the lithium-induced accumulation of IP_1 depends on the brain region and the strain (Savolainen et al. 1990). It seems problematic to use the results on the acute effect of lithium from in vitro experiments with brain slices to speculate on the mode of therapeutic action of lithium in vivo after long-term treatment.

Among the many receptors known to couple with phosphoinositide hydrolysis via G proteins, muscarinic cholinergic receptors have been of the greatest interest. Lithium-induced reduction of inositol and accumulation of IP_1 were shown to be reversed by coadministration of anticholinergic agents (Allison and Blisner 1976; Allison et al. 1976; Sherman et al. 1985) and synergistically enhanced by coadministration of cholinergic stimulants (Honchar et al. 1983, 1990; Sherman et al. 1986; Ackermann et al. 1987; Savolainen et al. 1988a,b; Whitworth et al. 1990). In these in vivo experiments, however, coadministration of lithium and cholinomimetics produces seizures, which themselves, in turn, potentially involve multiple signal-transduction systems, resulting in perturbation of phosphoinositide metabolism (Hirvonen et al. 1989; Jope et al. 1992). Therefore, the biochemical alterations observed in rats treated with lithium in combination with cholinomimetic agents should be interpreted with caution. Additionally, relatively high doses of lithium, which are often toxic rather than therapeutic doses, are necessary to alter the phosphoinositide hydrolysis system after short-term administration of lithium in vivo. Taken together with the notion that such an acute effect is not likely to explain fully its therapeutic efficacy, which is observed only after long-term administration, the effects on phosphoinositide metabolism described above may have more relevance to its toxic effect than to its therapeutic efficacy.

Thus, data from experiments with chronic, or at least subchronic, administration of lithium at therapeutically effective plasma concentrations are likely to provide the most relevant information to correlate the changes in phosphoinositide metabolism with the therapeutic action of lithium as an antimanic as well as a mood-stabilizing drug. Table 1 summarizes results that

TABLE 1. Effects of long-term administration of lithium on phosphoinositide turnover

Tissue	Lithium administration paradigm	Effects of lithium	Comments	References
Rat cortex	Dietary Li_2CO_3 for ~4 weeks	Increase in inositol monophosphatase activity		Renshaw et al. (1986)
Rat cortex	Dietary LiCl for 30 days	Attenuation of basal and noradrenaline-stimulated IP_1 accumulation		Casebolt and Jope (1987)
Rat cortex	Dietary Li_2CO_3 for 2 weeks	Attenuation of carbachol- and noradrenaline-stimulated IP_1 accumulation Enhancement of carbachol- and noradrenaline-stimulated IP_1 accumulation after withdrawal from lithium treatment	Acute LiCl administration attenuates carbachol-stimulated, but not noradrenaline-stimulated, IP_1 accumulation	Kendall and Nahorski (1987)
Rat cortex	LiCl i.p. or dietary Li_2CO_3 followed by LiCl i.p.	Unaltered inositol monophosphatase activity	Phosphoinositide levels are not altered	Honchar et al. (1989)
Rat cortex, hippocampus, and striatum	Dietary LiCl for 30 days	Attenuation of noradrenaline-stimulated IP_1 accumulation in all regions Attenuation of carbachol-stimulated IP_1 accumulation in striatum, but not in cortex or hippocampus Attenuation of 5-HT-stimulated IP_1 accumulation in hippocampus and striatum, but not in cortex	NaF-stimulated inositol phospholipid hydrolysis is unaltered	Casebolt and Jope (1989)

Rat cortex	LiCl s.c. for 3 and 16 days	Attenuation of 5-HT-, carbachol-, and noradrenaline-stimulated IP_1 accumulation Attenuation of NaF-stimulated IP_1 accumulation in membranes	Muscarinic cholinergic and 5-HT_2 binding is unaltered	Godfrey et al. (1989)
Rat cortex and striatum	Dietary LiCl for 13 days	Attenuation of carbachol-stimulated IP_1 accumulation following preincubation with 2.5 m*M* inositol in cortex, but not in striatum Increased inositol levels in cortex, but not in striatum	Without preincubation with inositol, carbachol-stimulated IP_1 accumulation is unaltered in both regions	Whitworth and Kendall (1989)
Rat cortex	Dietary LiCl for 10 days	Attenuation of 5-HT-stimulated IP_1 accumulation		Newman et al. (1990)
Rat hippocampus	Dietary LiCl for 3 weeks	Attenuation of noradrenaline-stimulated IP_1 accumulation Unaltered carbachol-stimulated IP_1 accumulation	5-HT-induced inhibition of carbachol-stimulated IP_1 accumulation is abolished by lithium administration	Newman et al. (1991b)
Rat cortex, hippocampus, and striatum (membranes)	Dietary LiCl for 4 weeks	Attenuation of carbachol-, GTPγS-, and NaF-stimulated PI hydrolysis		Song and Jope (1992)

GTP, guanosine triphosphate; IP_1, inositol monophosphate; PI, phosphatidylinositol.

can be interpreted as effects of long-term treatment with lithium, that are not simply effects of acutely administered lithium also seen after longer treatment. Although agonist-induced, receptor-mediated inositol phospholipid metabolism has been generally reported to be reduced by long-term treatment with lithium, the individual results are subtly inconsistent with each other in terms of affected receptors in discrete brain regions (Casebolt and Jope 1987, 1989; Kendall and Nahorski 1987; Godfrey et al. 1989). NaF-stimulated inositol phospholipid hydrolysis, which is thought to represent receptor-independent direct activation of G proteins associated with phosphoinositide turnover, has been reported to be attenuated (Godfrey et al. 1989) or unaltered (Casebolt and Jope 1989) after lithium treatment. Although the molecular mechanisms underlying alterations in phosphoinositide metabolism caused by long-term administration of lithium have not yet been elucidated, it is unlikely that a simple inositol depletion hypothesis can fully explain the results, and other mechanisms may be involved in the alterations caused by long-term lithium treatment.

Several studies have reported that the compositional ratio of phospholipids in plasma membranes is altered by long-term administration of lithium (Joseph et al. 1987; López-Corcuera et al. 1988; Navidi et al. 1991). Such alterations should lead to altered membrane fluidity (López-Corcuera et al. 1988), which may, in turn, affect the coupling efficacy between proteins that are involved in signal-transduction, thus resulting in altered cellular function.

In conclusion, the well-defined inhibitory action of lithium on inositol phospholipid metabolism in vitro or the inositol depletion hypothesis, based on the in vitro effect in conjunction with the results of experiments with short-term administration of lithium, cannot be applied directly to the situation in vivo, in which the clinical efficacy of lithium is apparent only after long-term administration. Further investigations are necessary to draw a conclusion concerning the relevance of inositol phospholipid metabolism to the therapeutic efficacy of lithium.

Adenylyl Cyclase System

Numerous studies have verified that lithium has a generally inhibitory effect in vitro on adenylyl cyclase activity and consequently on cyclic AMP production. However, the concentration of lithium necessary for such inhibition has varied according to the experimental conditions, such as the species and strain, the organs that the materials were derived from, the brain regions of interest when brain was chosen as the material, the material investigated (slice or membrane), the methods of membrane preparation, and the agonists or stimulants used. Although noradrenaline-stimulated accumulation of cyclic AMP in human brain slices was reported to be inhibited significantly by 1 m*M* lithium (Newman et al. 1983), higher concentrations of lithium have often been needed to demonstrate significant attenuation of adenylyl cyclase activity or cyclic AMP accumulation, and thus it has been generally accepted that the inhibitory in vitro effect of lithium on the adenylyl cyclase system has less relevance to its clinical therapeutic effectiveness than its effect on inositol phospholipid metabolism (Sillence and Downes 1992). Additionally, as discussed in the preceding section of this chapter, the ex vivo rather than in vitro effect of lithium, if any, should be considered to be associated with its therapeutic efficacy. In conjunction with the notion that the in vitro inhibitory effects of lithium on adenylyl cyclase activity stimulated by vasopressin (Dousa 1974; Dousa and Hechter 1970) and thyrotropin (Burke 1970; Wolff et al. 1970) should be mechanisms underlying its common side effects (Lenox and Manji 1995), namely, nephrogenic diabetes insipidus and subclinical hypothyroidism, respectively, the in vitro effects of lithium are likely to be involved in its toxic or adverse effects rather than its therapeutic or mood-stabilizing effects.

The changes in adenylyl cyclase systems in the central nervous system that have been reported in ex vivo experiments, i.e., in vitro measurement after long-term in vivo treatment, are listed in Table 2. Although the results are not necessarily consistent, components of the adenylyl cyclase system beyond the respective receptors, the interactions between these components, or both have been assumed to be the molecular sites of action of long-term lithium treatment in almost all studies.

Colin et al. (1991) reported that long-term treatment with lithium increased the levels of mRNA and protein for both calmodulin-sensitive (type 1) and calmodulin-insensitive (type 2) adenylyl cyclase in rat cerebral cortex. This quantitative change may underlie the increase in basal cyclic AMP or adenylyl cyclase activity that has been reported so far (Ebstein et al. 1980; Newman and Belmaker 1987). However, it should be noted that few reports have shown such increased basal activities and that other studies have reported no functional alteration or even a decrease in basal adenylyl cyclase activity.

In vivo microdialysis has demonstrated that long-term lithium treatment augments the basal level of extracellular cyclic AMP and reduces the noradrenaline-stimulated response expressed as a percentage of the corresponding basal value in the prefrontal cortex in vivo (Masana et al. 1991). In a subsequent investigation, the same authors ascribed the lithium-induced increase in the basal cyclic AMP level to inactivation of G_i function (Masana et al. 1992). On the other hand, Mørk and Geisler (1995) reported that administration of lithium for 4 weeks reduced the level of extracellular cyclic AMP in the dorsal hippocampus assessed by in vivo microdialysis after stimulation with noradrenaline and forskolin, leaving the baseline levels of cyclic AMP unaltered.

G Proteins

From the numerous biochemical and pharmacological studies on the effects of lithium on the major two signal-transduction systems, i.e., phosphoinositide turnover and adenylyl cyclase, as described above, it appears evident that the postulated site of action of the ion lies beyond the respective neurotransmitter

TABLE 2. Effects of long-term administration of lithium on adenylyl cyclase systems

Tissue and preparation	Stimulants	Effects of lithium (postulated site of action)	References
Slices			
Rat cortex	Noradrenaline	Attenuation	Ebstein et al. (1980)
Rat cerebellum	Noradrenaline	No alteration	Schultz et al. (1981)
Rat cortex	Noradrenaline	No alteration	Andersen et al. (1984a)
Rat cortex	2-Chloroadenosine	No alteration	Newman et al. (1984)
	Noradrenaline	No alteration	
Mouse cortex	Noradrenaline	No alteration	Hamburger-Bar et al. (1986)
	Forskolin	No alteration	
	2-Chloroadenosine	Attenuation only in 2 of 6 strains	
Rat striatum	Dopamine	No alteration	Whitworth and Kendall (1989)
	Carbachol (inhibition)	No alteration (enhanced inhibition in vitro)	
Membranes			
Rat olfactory tubercle, striatum, and cortex	Dopamine	No alteration	Geisler and Klysner (1978)
Rat cerebellum	Noradrenaline	No alteration	Türck et al. (1981)
Rat striatum	Dopamine	No alteration	Staunton et al. (1982)
Rat cortex	Fluoride	No alteration	Andersen and Geisler (1984)
	Forskolin	Attenuation (catalytic unit)	
Rat cortex	Forskolin	Attenuation (catalytic unit)	Andersen et al. (1984c)
Rat cortex and limbic forebrain	Fluoride	No alteration	Andersen et al. (1984b)
Rat striatum and olfactory tubercle	Dopamine	No alteration	Geisler and Klysner (1985)
	Fluoride	No alteration	
Rat hippocampus	5-HT	Augmentation	Hotta and Yamawaki (1986)
	GTP	Attenuation	

Rat cortex	Ca^{2+}-calmodulin	Attenuation	Mørk and Geisler (1987)
	GTP	No alteration (catalytic unit)	
Rat cortex	Fluoride	No alteration	Newman and Belmaker (1987)
	Manganese	Attenuation	
	Forskolin	No alteration	
	Isoproterenol	Attenuation	
	GppNHp	Attenuation (G_s or catalytic unit)	
Rat striatum	Dopamine	No alteration	
	Forskolin	No alteration	
	met-Enkephalin (inhibition)	No alteration	
Rat cortex	Noradrenaline	Dependent on GTP concentration	Mørk and Geisler (1989a)
Rat striatum	Dopamine	(G protein or receptor/G protein	
Rat hippocampus	5-HT	coupling)	
Rat cortex	Forskolin	Attenuation (G protein or catalytic unit)	Mørk and Geisler (1989c)
Rat hippocampus	Ca^{2+}-calmodulin	Augmentation	Mørk and Geisler (1989b)
	5-HT (inhibition)	Attenuation (G_i protein)	
Rat striatum	Ca^{2+}-calmodulin	Attenuation	
	GTP (inhibition)	No alteration	
Rat hippocampus	5-HT (inhibition)	Attenuation	Newman et al. (1990)
Rat hippocampus	Carbachol (inhibition)	Attenuation (G_i protein)	Newman et al. (1991a,b)
Rat cortex	Isoproterenol	Attenuation	Odagaki et al. (1991c)
	GppNHp	No alteration (β-adrenoceptor or receptor/G protein coupling)	
Rat hippocampus	5-HT (inhibition)	No alteration	Odagaki et al. (1991b)
	GppNHp (inhibition)	No alteration	

GppNHp, guanylylimidodiphosphate; GTP, guanosine triphosphate.

receptors. In this context, the trimeric transducing G proteins are of great interest, since G proteins are involved in both transmembrane signaling pathways and play a pivotal role as transducers as well as amplifiers of the signals. Although several lines of studies have provided indirect evidence that G proteins are targets of the therapeutic action of lithium, few studies provided direct evidence about the relationship between G proteins and the action of lithium until the late 1980s. In 1988, Avissar et al. reported that isoproterenol- and carbachol-stimulated increases in [^{3}H]guanosine triphosphate (GTP) binding in rat cortical membranes were inhibited by lithium at therapeutically relevant concentrations in both in vitro and ex vivo experiments. This finding means that lithium interferes functionally with the receptor-associated G proteins or with receptor–G-protein coupling, because basal unstimulated GTP binding is not altered by lithium at all. Later studies by the same investigators showed that the in vitro effect of lithium was reversed by Mg^{2+} (Avissar et al. 1991) and that the in vitro and ex vivo effects of the ion were observed preferentially in the central nervous system as compared with peripheral (cardiac ventricle) tissues (Schreiber et al. 1990). On the basis of these results, in conjunction with other studies in animals (Avissar et al. 1990) and clinical investigations using mononuclear leukocyte membranes (Schreiber et al. 1991), they developed a novel hypothesis that hyperfunctional G proteins underlie the pathophysiology of bipolar affective disorders (Avissar and Schreiber 1992). Although their G-protein hyperfunction hypothesis looks very attractive, the effects of lithium on G proteins are still controversial (Table 3). By using GTPγS release as an indicator of G-protein function, Ellis and Lenox (1991) showed that lithium in vitro altered neither the G proteins coupled with α_2-adrenoceptors in human platelets nor those coupled with muscarinic acetylcholine receptors in rat cardiac ventricle. Similar negative results were obtained recently by means of another functional characteristic intrinsic to G proteins, GTP-hydrolyzing activity (Odagaki et al. 1997). Furthermore, complete abolition of receptor-coupled G-protein function by lithium, as shown by Avissar and colleagues, should lead to null responses in second-messenger systems transduced via the G proteins, which is inconsistent with the numerous previous reports that lithium inhibits both phosphoinositide turnover and adenylyl cyclase, but far from completely abolishing them. It should be noticed, however, that only in vitro effects of lithium, mainly on the G_i family associated with adenylyl cyclase inhibition, were investigated in latter two studies.

Several laboratories have reported the quantitative effects of long-term lithium treatment on G proteins (Table 3). Although the administration of lithium generally results in a decrease in the mRNAs for the α subunits of G protein (Colin et al. 1991; Li et al. 1991), the results on alterations in protein levels after lithium treatment have been inconsistent. Colin et al. (1991) reported decreased $G_{i1/2\alpha}$ levels in the cortex, whereas others have reported no alterations (Hsiao et al. 1992; Masana et al. 1992) or even increased $G_{i\alpha}$ in some discrete brain regions (Lesch et al. 1991). Then, G proteins may be

TABLE 3. Effects of lithium on G proteins

Measure	Tissue	Lithium administration paradigm	Effects of lithium	References
mRNA	Rat cortex	Dietary LiCl for 21 days	Decrease in mRNAs for $G_{s\alpha}$, $G_{i1\alpha}$, and $G_{i2\alpha}$	Li et al. (1991)
	Rat cortex	Dietary Li_2CO_3 for 4 weeks	Decrease in mRNAs for $G_{i1\alpha}$ and $G_{i2\alpha}$ Unaltered mRNAs for $G_{s\alpha}$, $G_{o\alpha}$, and G_{β}	Colin et al. (1991)
Protein level	Rat cortex	Dietary Li_2CO_3 for 4 weeks	Decrease in $G_{i1/2\alpha}$ No alteration in G_{β}	Colin et al. (1991)
	Rat brain regions	Dietary Li_2CO_3 for 21 days	Increase in $G_{i\alpha}$ (hippocampus and hypothalamus) No alteration in $G_{s\alpha}$ or $G_{o\alpha}$	Lesch et al. (1991)
	Human platelet	Li_2CO_3 orally for 14 days	No alteration in $G_{i2\alpha}$	Hsiao et al. (1992)
	Rat cortex	Dietary Li_2CO_3 for 4–5 weeks	No alteration in $G_{s\alpha}$ or $G_{i1/2\alpha}$	Masana et al. (1992)
Bacterial toxin-catalyzed ADP-ribosylation	Human platelet	Li_2CO_3 orally for 10–188 days	Increase in IAP-sensitive ADP-ribosylation after withdrawal from lithium for 16–30 days in patients with bipolar affective disorder	Watanabe et al. (1990)
	Rat cardiac ventricle, aorta, and partially purified G_i	In vitro	Attenuation of IAP-sensitive ADP-ribosylation	Kawamoto et al. (1991) Watanabe et al. (1991)
	Rat cortex and hippocampus	Dietary Li_2CO_3 for 3 weeks and in vitro	No alteration in IAP-sensitive ADP-ribosylation	Odagaki et al. (1991a)
	Human platelet	Li_2CO_3 orally for 14 days	Increase in IAP-sensitive ADP-ribosylation Unaltered cholera toxin-sensitive ADP-ribosylation	Hsiao et al. (1992)
	Rat cortex	Dietary Li_2CO_3 for 4–5 weeks	Increase in IAP-sensitive ADP-ribosylation Unaltered cholera toxin-sensitive ADP-ribosylation	Masana et al. (1992)
GTP binding	Rat cortex	Li_2CO_3 i.p. for 12–21 days and in vitro	Inhibition of isoproterenol- and carbachol-stimulated increases	Avissar et al. (1988)
	PC12 cells cultured with nerve growth factor	In vitro	Increase in maximum binding	Volonté (1988)
GTPγS release	Human platelet and rat cardiac ventricle	In vitro	No alteration in adrenaline-stimulated increase in platelet or carbachol-stimulated increase in cardiac ventricle	Ellis and Lenox (1991)
GTP hydrolysis	Human platelet, rat hippocampus and striatum	In vitro	No alteration in adrenaline-stimulated increase in platelet or agonist-induced increase in brain regions	Odagaki et al. (1997)

ADP, adenosine diphosphate; IAP, islet-activating protein

regulated subtly and differentially, depending on the region of the brain and the lithium treatment regimen. It remains to be elucidated whether such alterations have relevance to the functional role of the G proteins associated with the respective receptor subtypes.

Bacterial toxins, such as cholera and pertussis toxin, have been used in many investigations of G proteins. An increase in pertussis toxin (islet-activating protein, IAP)-sensitive adenosine diphosphate (ADP)-ribosylation has been reported after administration of lithium in rat cortex (Masana et al. 1992) and human platelets (Hsiao et al. 1992). Even though there is no alteration in protein levels, they consider such changes responsible for the increased basal cyclic AMP accumulation that has sometimes been reported after long-term treatment with lithium. On the other hand, IAP-sensitive ADP-ribosylation has been reported to be inhibited by lithium at therapeutically relevant concentrations in vitro (Kawamoto et al. 1991; Watanabe et al. 1991). However, the authors were unable to detect any alteration in IAP-sensitive ADP-ribosylation in rat brain membranes in vitro or ex vivo (Odagaki et al. 1991a).

Although G proteins are likely candidates for sites of action of lithium, further studies are necessary to elucidate fully the relevance of G proteins to the therapeutic effectiveness of lithium and the pathophysiology of affective disorders (Manji 1992; Spiegel et al. 1992). In particular, functional studies of the ex vivo effects of lithium on the G proteins coupled with the respective receptors associated with adenylyl cyclase stimulation (G_s) and inositol phospholipid metabolism (G_p) are awaited.

Protein Phosphorylation and Gene Expression

With the rapid progress in molecular biology in the last decade, evidence has accumulated that the expression of mRNA for various substances is altered by lithium treatment (see Jope and Williams 1994; Manji and Lenox 1994; Manji et al. 1995, 1996). The effects of long-term lithium administration on the levels of mRNA for G-protein subclasses have been mentioned previously (Table 3). Such alteration is of great interest when the pivotal role of G proteins in multiple signal-transduction systems is considered. Lithium has also been reported to alter the mRNA levels for a number of substances that have been known to play critical roles in modulating signal-transduction systems and thus cellular function at discrete steps and by varied means, such as adenylyl cyclase types 1 and 2 (Colin et al. 1991), neuropeptide Y (Weiner et al. 1992), and glucocorticoid receptor (Peiffer et al. 1991). The expression of mRNA for c-fos, an immediate early gene product that is known to be induced by many stimuli, has been reported to be augmented by lithium treatment (Arenander et al. 1989; Kalasapudi et al. 1990; Divish et al. 1991; Weiner et al. 1991), especially when induced by stimulants related to activation of protein kinase C (PKC). Because c-fos is a transcription factor regulating the expression of secondary genes, such changes in c-fos expression induced by lithium treatment may underlie the alteration in the expression of other genes described above.

PKC is a ubiquitous enzyme that plays a crucial role in the regulation of transcriptional and posttranscriptional processes. In view of the findings noted above concerning gene expression, it seems plausible that the multifarious effects of lithium result from its action on PKC and/or cellular events mediated by this enzyme. There is substantial experimental evidence that lithium affects PKC and PKC-mediated responses (reviewed by Manji and Lenox 1994). Lithium facilitates a number of short-term PKC-mediated responses by mimicking the action of phorbol ester and down-regulates PKC, leading to an attenuation of phorbol ester-mediated responses after long-term treatment. The down-regulation of PKC is time dependent and is selective for different isoenzymes (α and ε) in particular brain regions (the hippocampus subiculum and CA_1 regions) (Manji et al. 1993, 1996). In line with the notion described above, Lenox and associates make much account of the reduction of myristoylated alanine-rich C kinase substrate (MARCKS), a prominent and preferential substrate in the brain for PKC, after long-term treatment with lithium as a likely molecular target for its therapeutic action (Lenox et al. 1992; Watson and Lenox, 1996; Lenox et al. 1996). The reduction of MARCKS protein by lithium was antagonized by inositol, suggesting that lithium-induced inositol depletion underlies the phenomenon. Interestingly, the reduction of MARCKS protein also occurs when the cells are treated with valproate but not with carbamazepine, probably through a mechanism different from that in the case of lithium-induced reduction (Lenox et al. 1996).

Whatever the mechanism(s) involved in the alterations in PKC-related events as well as gene expression exemplified above, these alterations are of considerable interest, because the time lag necessary for the occurrence of such alterations during lithium exposure conveniently explains the delay in the response to lithium treatment seen in clinical practice. Further studies on the effects of lithium on genetic expression and the underlying molecular mechanisms will help elucidate the pathogenesis of affective disorders.

Conclusion

Lithium remains the primary drug for the treatment of patients with bipolar affective disorders because of its antimanic as well as its prophylactic effects. Despite its structural simplicity as a monovalent cation and abundant biochemical, pharmacological, and electrophysiological data on its potential effects in animal and clinical experiments, the molecular mechanisms or sites of action of the therapeutic efficacy of lithium are not fully understood. Although lithium appears to affect signal-transduction systems, at multiple sites and in various ways, it is difficult to determine which alterations are relevant to its therapeutic action. It is likely that the therapeutic effects of lithium are caused by the altered responsiveness of cellular function to external stimuli that results from integration of the respective changes. In this context, synaptic plasticity after long-term lithium administration based on protein phosphorylation and gene expression should be considered. Of course, the significance of the inositol-depletion hypothesis has not been impaired, since the depletion of inositol acutely induced by lithium must play an important role in initiating the subsequent cellular adaptive changes, although the therapeutic efficacy of lithium cannot be explained simply by the hypothesis.

Although it is beyond the scope of this article to review the modes of action of psychotropic drugs (e.g., carbamazepine, valproate, clonazepam, calcium antagonists) and treatments (e.g., electroconvulsive therapy) other than lithium that are effective against manic-depressive illness, it is of considerable interest to explore the sites of action that these treatments may share with lithium. Dopamine- and noradrenaline-stimulated adenylyl cyclase activity in rat and mouse cerebral cortical membranes was inhibited in vitro in a concentration-dependent manner by carbamazepine (Palmer 1979). The reduced formation of inositol phosphate in response to 5-HT, carbachol, and noradrenaline seen after long-term treatment with lithium (Elphick et al. 1988; Godfrey et al. 1989) did not occur with carbamazepine in vitro or ex vivo (Elphick et al. 1988). The effects of lithium on G-protein function are shared by carbamazepine as well as by electroconvulsive shock (Avissar et al. 1990). On the other hand, Lesch et al. (1991) have reported that the quantity of G-protein α subunits is regulated differentially by long-term lithium and carbamazepine treatment. Treatment of PC12 cells with carbamazepine was shown to inhibit the expression of c-fos induced by cyclic AMP-dependent pathways without affecting expression induced by the activation of PKC, whereas lithium treatment augmented only PKC-mediated expression of c-fos (Divish et al. 1991). Reduction of the expression of MARCKS protein in cultured cells also occured after valproate treatment probably by a mechanism different from that in the case of lithium-induced alteration, but not after carbamazepine administration (Lenox et al. 1996).

As mentioned previously, plasma-membrane fluidity has been reported to be altered by long-term lithium treatment (López-Corcuera et al. 1988). Whatever the mechanisms involved in this change, such an alteration should result in changes in the function of the proteins that constitute the signal-transduction system, as well as in the functional coupling efficacy between them. Thus, not only biochemical, pharmacological, and electrophysiological, but also biophysical investigations may be necessary to elucidate fully the mechanism of action of lithium.

Although lithium is an efficacious drug for bipolar affective disorders, it is far from ideal, owing to many troublesome problems. For example, 20%–30% of patients with bipolar affective disorders do not respond to lithium treatment. Furthermore, even if it works well, there is a lag time of days or even weeks in the onset of its effectiveness, and toxic and adverse effects should always be taken into consideration. Full elucidation of the effects of lithium in the future may lead to the development of a novel drug with more efficacy and fewer toxic and adverse effects and to a better understanding of the pathophysiology of bipolar affective disorders.

References

Ackermann KE, Gish BG, Honchar MP, Sherman WR (1987) Evidence that inositol 1-phosphate in brain of lithium-treated rats results mainly from phosphatidylinositol metabolism. Biochem J 242:517–524

Allison JH, Blisner ME (1976) Inhibition of the effect of lithium on brain inositol by atropine and scopolamine. Biochem Biophys Res Commun 68:1332–1338

Allison JH, Stewart MA (1971) Reduced brain inositol in lithium-treated rats. Nature New Biol 233:267–268

Allison JH, Blisner ME, Holland WH, Hipps PP, Sherman WR (1976) Increased brain myo-inositol 1-phosphate in lithium-treated rats. Biochem Biophys Res Commun 71:664–670

Andersen PH, Geisler A (1984) Lithium inhibition of forskolin-stimulated adenylate cyclase. Neuropsychobiology 12:1–3

Andersen PH, Geisler A, Klysner R (1984a) No change in rat cerebral cortex calmodulin content following chronic treatment with lithium, reserpine, imipramine, and lithium combined with reserpine or imipramine. Acta Pharmacol Toxicol 54:394–399

Andersen PH, Klysner R, Geisler A (1984b) Fluoride-stimulated adenylate cyclase activity in rat brain following chronic treatment with psychotropic drugs. Neuropharmacology 23:445–447

Andersen PH, Klysner R, Geisler A (1984c) Forskolin-stimulated adenylate cyclase activity in rat cerebral cortex following chronic treatment with psychotropic drugs. Acta Pharmacol Toxicol 55:278–282

Arenander AT, de Vellis J, Herschman HR (1989) Induction of c-fos and TIS genes in cultured rat astrocytes by neurotransmitters. J Neurosci Res 24:107–114

Attwood PV, Ducep J-B, Chanal M-C (1988) Purification and properties of myo-inositol-1-phosphatase from bovine brain. Biochem J 253:387–394

Avissar S, Schreiber G (1992) The involvement of guanine nucleotide binding proteins in the pathogenesis and treatment of affective disorders. Biol Psychiatr 31:435–459

Avissar S, Schreiber G, Danon A, Belmaker RH (1988) Lithium inhibits adrenergic and cholinergic increases in GTP binding in rat cortex. Nature 331:440–442

Avissar S, Schreiber G, Aulakh CS, Wozniak KM, Murphy DL (1990) Carbamazepine and electroconvulsive shock attenuate β-adrenoceptor and muscarinic cholinoceptor coupling to G proteins in rat cortex. Eur J Pharmacol (Mol Pharmacol Sec) 189:99–103

Avissar S, Murphy DL, Schreiber G (1991) Magnesium reversal of lithium inhibition of β-adrenergic and muscarinic receptor coupling to G proteins. Biochem Pharmacol 41:171–175

Baraban JM, Worley PF, Snyder SH (1989) Second messenger systems and psychoactive drug action: focus on the phosphoinositide system and lithium. Am J Psychiatr 146:1251–1260

Batty I, Nahorski SR (1985) Differential effects of lithium on muscarinic receptor stimulation of inositol phosphates in rat cerebral cortex slices. J Neurochem 45:1514–1521

Batty I, Nahorski SR (1987) Lithium inhibits muscarinic-receptor-stimulated inositol tetrakisphosphate accumulation in rat cerebral cortex. Biochem J 247:797–800

Berridge MJ, Downes CP, Hanley MR (1982) Lithium amplifies agonist-dependent phosphatidylinositol responses in brain and salivary glands. Biochem J 206:587–595

Berridge MJ, Downes CP, Hanley MR (1989) Neural and developmental actions of lithium: a unifying hypothesis. Cell 59:411–419

Birnbaumer L (1992) Receptor-to-effector signaling through G proteins: roles for βγ dimers as well as α subunits. Cell 71:1069–1072

Birnbaumer L, Abramowitz J, Brown AM (1990) Receptor-effector coupling by G proteins. Biochim Biophys Acta 1031:163–224

Brami BA, Leli U, Hauser G (1993) Elevated phosphatidyl-CMP is not the source of diacylglycerol accumulation induced by lithium in NG108-15 cells. J Neurochem 60:1137–1142

Burke G (1970) Effects of cations and ouabain on thyroid adenyl cyclase. Biochim Biophys Acta 220:30–41

Casebolt TL, Jope RS (1987) Chronic lithium treatment reduces norepinephrine-stimulated inositol phospholipid hydrolysis in rat cortex. Eur J Pharmacol 140:245–246

Casebolt TL, Jope RS (1989) Long-term lithium treatment selectively reduces receptor-coupled inositol phospholipid hydrolysis in rat brain. Biol Psychiatr 25: 329–340

Colin SF, Chang H-C, Mollner S, Pfeuffer T, Reed RR, Duman RS, Nestler EJ (1991) Chronic lithium regulates the expression of adenylate cyclase and G_i-protein α subunit in rat cerebral cortex. Proc Natl Acad Sci USA 88:10634–10637

Dixon JF, Lee CH, Los GV, Hokin LE (1992) Lithium enhances accumulation of [^{3}H]inositol radioactivity and mass of second messenger inositol 1,4,5-trisphosphate in monkey cerebral cortex slices. J Neurochem 59:2332–2335

Divish MM, Sheftel G, Boyle A, Kalasapudi VD, Papolos DF, Lachman HM (1991) Differential effect of lithium on fos protooncogene expression mediated by receptor and postreceptor activators of protein kinase C and cyclic adenosine monophosphate: model for its antimanic action. J Neurosci Res 28:40–48

Dousa TP (1974) Interaction of lithium with vasopressin-sensitive cyclic AMP system of human renal medulla. Endocrinology 95:1359–1366

Dousa T, Hechter O (1970) The effect of NaCl and LiCl on vasopressin-sensitive adenyl cyclase. Life Sci 9:765–770

Drummond AH (1987) Lithium and inositol-linked signalling mechanisms. Trends Pharmacol Sci 8:129–133

Ebstein RP, Hermoni M, Belmaker RH (1980) The effect of lithium on noradrenaline-induced cyclic AMP accumulation in rat brain: inhibition after chronic treatment and absence of supersensitivity. J Pharmacol Exp Ther 213:161–167

Ellis J, Lenox RH (1991) Receptor coupling to G proteins: interactions not affected by lithium. Lithium 2:141–147

Elphick M, Taghavi Z, Powell T, Godfrey PP (1988) Alteration of inositol phospholipid metabolism in rat cortex by lithium but not carbamazepine. Eur J Pharmacol 156:411–414

Gee NS, Ragan CI, Watling KJ, Aspley S, Jackson RG, Reid GG, Gani D, Shute JK (1988a) The purification and properties of myo-inositol monophosphatase from bovine brain. Biochem J 249:883–889

Gee NS, Reid GG, Jackson RG, Barnaby RJ, Ragan CI (1988b) Purification and properties of inositol-1,4-bisphosphatase from bovine brain. Biochem J 253:777–782

Geisler A, Klysner R (1978) Influence of lithium on dopamine-stimulated adenylate cyclase activity in rat brain. Life Sci 23:635–636

Geisler A, Klysner R (1985) The effect of lithium in vitro and in vivo on dopamine-sensitive adenylate cyclase activity in dopaminergic areas of the rat brain. Acta Pharmacol Toxicol 56:1–5

Gilman AG (1987) G proteins: transducers of receptor-generated signals. Annu Rev Biochem 56:615–649

Godfrey PP (1989) Potentiation by lithium of CMP-phospatidate formation in carbachol-stimulated rat cerebral-cortical slices and its reversal by myo-inositol. Biochem J 258:621–624

Godfrey PP, McClue SJ, White AM, Wood AJ, Grahame-Smith DG (1989) Sub-acute and chronic in vivo lithium treatment inhibits agonist- and sodium fluoride-stimulated inositol phosphate production in rat cortex. J Neurochem 52:498–506

Gudermann T, Schöneberg T, Schultz G (1997) Functional and structural complexity of signal transduction via G-protein-coupled receptors. Annu Rev Neurosci 20:399–427

Hallcher LM, Sherman WR (1980) The effects of lithium ion and other agents on the activity of myo-inositol-1-phosphatase from bovine brain. J Biol Chem 255:10896–10901

Hamburger-Bar R, Robert M, Newman M, Belmaker RH (1986) Interstrain correlation between behavioural effects of lithium and effects on cortical cyclic AMP. Pharmacol Biochem Behav 24:9–13

Heacock AM, Seguin EB, Agranoff BW (1993) Measurement of receptor-activated phosphoinositide turnover in rat brain: nonequivalence of inositol phosphate and CDP-diacylglycerol formation. J Neurochem 60:1087–1092

Hepler JR, Gilman AG (1992) G proteins. Trends Biol Sci 17:383–387

Hirvonen M-R, Savolainen K (1991) Lithium-induced decrease of brain inositol and increase of brain inositol-1-phosphate is transient. Neurochem Res 16:905–911

Hirvonen M-R, Komulainen H, Paljärvi L, Savolainen K (1989) Time-course of malaoxon-induced alterations in brain regional inositol-1-phosphate levels in convulsing and nonconvulsing rats. Neurochem Res 14:143–147

Honchar MP, Olney JW, Sherman WR (1983) Systemic cholinergic agents induce seizures and brain damage in lithium-treated rats. Science 220:323–325

Honchar MP, Ackermann KE, Sherman WR (1989) Chronically administered lithium alters neither myo-inositol monophosphatase activity nor phosphoinositide levels in rat brain. J Neurochem 53:590–594

Honchar MP, Vogler GP, Gish BG, Sherman WR (1990) Evidence that phosphoinositide metabolism in rat cerebral cortex stimulated by pilocarpine, physostigmine, and pargyline in vivo is not changed by chronic lithium treatment. J Neurochem 55:1521–1525

Hotta I, Yamawaki S (1986) Lithium decreases 5-HT_1 receptors but increases 5-HT-sensitive adenylate cyclase activity in rat hippocampus. Biol Psychiatr 21:1382–1390

Hsiao JK, Manji HK, Chen G, Bitran JA, Risby ED, Potter WZ (1992) Lithium administration modulates platelet G_i in humans. Life Sci 50:227–233

Inhorn RC, Majerus PW (1987) Inositol polyphosphate 1-phosphatase from calf brain. J Biol Chem 262:15946–15952

Iñiguez-Lluhi J, Kleuss C, Gilman AG (1993) The importance of G-protein $\beta\gamma$ subunits. Trends Cell Biol 3:230–236

Jope RS, Williams MB (1994) Lithium and brain signal transduction systems. Biochem Pharmacol 47:429–441

Jope RS, Song L, Kolasa K (1992) Inositol trisphosphate, cyclic AMP, and cyclic GMP in rat brain regions after lithium and seizures. Biol Psychiatr 31:505–514

Joseph NE, Renshaw PF, Leigh JS Jr (1987) Systemic lithium administration alters rat cerebral cortex phospholipids. Biol Psychiatr 22:540–544

Kalasapudi VD, Sheftel G, Divish MM, Papolos DF, Lachman HM (1990) Lithium augments fos protooncogene expression in PC12 pheochromocytoma cells: implications for therapeutic action of lithium. Brain Res 521:47–54

Kawamoto H, Watanabe Y, Imaizumi T, Iwasaki T, Yoshida H (1991) Effects of lithium ion on ADP ribosylation of inhibitory GTP-binding protein by pertussis toxin, islet-activating protein. Eur J Pharmacol (Mol Pharmacol Sec) 206:33–37

Kendall DA, Nahorski SR (1987) Acute and chronic lithium treatments influence agonist and depolarization-stimulated inositol phospholipid hydrolysis in rat cerebral cortex. J Pharmacol Exp Ther 241:1023–1027

Kendall DA, Whitworth P (1990) Lithium amplifies inhibitions of inositol phospholipid hydrolysis in mammalian brain slices. Br J Pharmacol 100:723–728

Kennedy ED, Challis RAJ, Nahorski SR (1989) Lithium reduces the accumulation of inositol polyphosphate second messengers following cholinergic stimulation of cerebral cortex slices. J Neurochem 53:1652–1655

Kennedy ED, Challis RAJ, Raga CI, Nahorski SR (1990) Reduced inositol polyphosphate accumulation and inositol supply induced by lithium in stimulated cerebral cortex slices. Biochem J 267:781–786

Lee CH, Dixon JF, Reichman M, Moummi C, Los G, Hokin LE (1992) Li^+ increases accumulation of inositol 1,4,5-trisphosphate and inositol 1,3,4,5-tetrakisphosphate in cholinergically stimulated brain cortex slices in guinea pig, mouse and rat. Biochem J 282:377–385

Lenox HR, Manji HK (1995) Lithium. In: Schatzberg AF, Nemeroff CB (eds) Textbook of psychopharmacology. American Psychiatric Press, Washington, DC, pp 303–349

Lenox RH, Watson DG, Patel J, Ellis J (1992) Chronic lithium administration alters a prominent PKC substrate in rat hippocampus. Brain Res 570:333–340

Lenox RH, McNamara RK, Watterson JM, Watson DG (1996) Myristoylated alanine-rich C kinase substrate (MARCKS): a molecular target for the therapeutic action of mood stabilizers in the brain? J Clin Psychiatr 57 (suppl 13):23–31

Lesch KP, Aulakh CS, Tolliver TJ, Hill JL, Wolozin BL, Murphy DL (1991) Differential effects of long-term lithium and carbamazepine administration on $G_{s\alpha}$ and $G_{i\alpha}$ protein in rat brain. Eur J Pharmacol (Mol Pharmacol Sec) 207:355–359

Li PP, Tam Y-K, Young LT, Warsh JJ (1991) Lithium decreases Gs, Gi-1 and Gi-2 α-subunit mRNA levels in rat cortex. Eur J Pharmacol (Mol Pharmacol Sec) 206:165–166

López-Corcuera B, Giménez C, Aragón C (1988) Change of synaptic membrane lipid composition and fluidity by chronic administration of lithium. Biochim Biophys Acta 939:467–475

Manji HK (1992) G proteins: implications for psychiatry. Am J Psychiatr 149:746–760

Manji HK, Lenox RH (1994) Long-term action of lithium: a role for transcriptional and posttranscriptional factors regulated by protein kinase C. Synapse 16:11–28

Manji HK, Etcheberrigaray R, Chen G, Olds JL (1993) Lithium decreases membrane-associated protein kinase C in hippocampus: selectivity for the α isozyme. J Neurochem 61:2303–2310

Manji HK, Potter WZ, Lenox RH (1995) Signal transduction pathways. Molecular targets for lithium's action. Arch Gen Psychiatr 52:531–543

Manji HK, Chen G, Hsiao JK, Risby ED, Masana MI, Potter WZ (1996) Regulation of signal transduction pathways by mood-stabilizing agents: implications for the delayed onset of therapeutic efficacy. J Clin Psychiatr 57(suppl 13):34–46

Masana MI, Bitran JA, Hsiao JK, Mefford IN, Potter WZ (1991) Lithium effects on noradrenergic-linked adenylate cyclase activity in intact rat brain: an in vivo microdialysis study. Brain Res 538:333–336

Masana MI, Bitran JA, Hsiao JK, Potter WZ (1992) In vivo evidence that lithium inactivates G_i modulation of adenylate cyclase in brain. J Neurochem 59:200–205

Mørk A, Geisler A (1987) Effects of lithium on calmodulin-stimulated adenylate cyclase activity in cortical membranes from rat brain. Pharmacol Toxicol 60:17–23

Mørk A, Geisler A (1989a) Effects of GTP on hormone-stimulated adenylate cyclase activity in cerebral cortex, striatum, and hippocampus from rats treated chronically with lithium. Biol Psychiatr 26:279–288

Mørk A, Geisler A (1989b) Effects of lithium ex vivo on the GTP-mediated inhibition of calcium-stimulated adenylate cyclase activity in rat brain. Eur J Pharmacol 168:347–354

Mørk A, Geisler A (1989c) The effects of lithium in vitro and ex vivo on adenylate cyclase in brain are exerted by distinct mechanisms. Neuropharmacology 28:307–311

Mørk A, Geisler A (1995) Effects of chronic lithium treatment on agonist-enhanced extracellular concentrations of cyclic AMP in the dorsal hippocampus of freely moving rats. J Neurochem 65:134–139

Nahorski SR, Ragan CI, Challis RAJ (1991) Lithium and the phosphoinositide cycle: an example of uncompetitive inhibition and its pharmacological consequences. Trends Pharmacol Sci 12:297–303

Navidi M, Yoa F-G, Sun GY (1991) Brief chronic effects of lithium administration on rat brain phosphoinositides and phospholipids. J Neurosci Res 28:428–433

Newman ME, Belmaker RH (1987) Effects of lithium in vitro and ex vivo on components of the adenylate cyclase system in membranes from the cerebral cortex of the rat. Neuropharmacology 26:211–217

Newman M, Klein E, Birmaher B, Feinsod M, Belmaker RH (1983) Lithium at therapeutic concentrations inhibits human brain noradrenaline-sensitive cyclic AMP accumulation. Brain Res 278:380–381

Newman M, Zohar J, Kalian M, Belmaker RH (1984) The effects of chronic lithium and ECT on A_1 and A_2 adenosine receptor systems in rat brain. Brain Res 291:188–192

Newman ME, Drummer D, Lerer B (1990) Single and combined effects of desipramine and lithium on serotonergic receptor number and second messenger function in rat brain. J Pharmacol Exp Ther 252:826–831

Newman ME, Ben-Zeev A, Lerer B (1991a) Chloroamphetamine did not prevent the effects of chronic antidepressants on 5-hydroxytryptamine inhibition of forskolin-stimulated adenylate cyclase in rat hippocampus. Eur J Pharmacol (Mol Pharmacol Sec) 207:209–213

Newman ME, Shapira B, Lerer B (1991b) Effects of lithium and desipramine on second messenger responses in rat hippocampus: relation to G protein effects. Neuropharmacology 30:1297–1301

Odagaki Y, Koyama T, Yamashita I (1991a) Lithium does not alter ADP-ribosylation of Gi/Go catalyzed by pertussis toxin in rat brain. Pharmacol Toxicol 69:355–360

Odagaki Y, Koyama T, Yamashita I (1991b) No alterations in the 5-HT_{1A}-mediated inhibition of forskolin-stimulated adenylate cyclase activity in the hippocampal membranes from rats chronically treated with lithium or antidepressants. J Neural Transm 86:85–96

Odagaki Y, Koyama T, Matsubara S, Matsubara R, Yamashita I (1991c) Effects of lithium on β-adrenergic receptor-adenylate cyclase system in rat cerebral cortical membranes. Jpn J Pharmacol 55:407–414

Odagaki Y, Nishi N, Koyama T (1997) Lack of interfering effects of lithium on receptor/G protein coupling in human platelet and rat brain membranes. Biol Psychiatr 42:697–703

Palmer GC (1979) Interactions of antiepileptic drugs on adenylate cyclase and phosphodiesterases in rat and mouse cerebrum. Exp Neurol 63:322–335

Peiffer A, Veilleux S, Barden N (1991) Antidepressant and other centrally acting drugs regulate glucocorticoid receptor messenger RNA levels in rat brain. Psychoneuroendocrinology 16:505–515

Rana R, Hokin LE (1990) Role of phosphoinositides in transmembrane signaling. Physiol Rev 70:115–164

Renshaw PF, Joseph NE, Leigh JS Jr (1986) Chronic dietary lithium induces increased levels of myo-inositol-1-phosphatase activity in rat cerebral cortex homogenates. Brain Res 380:401–404

Savolainen KM, Nelson SR, Samson FE, Pazdernik TL (1988a) Soman-induced convulsions affect the inositol lipid signaling system: potentiation by lithium; attenuation by atropine and diazepam. Toxicol Appl Pharmacol 96:305–314

Savolainen KM, Terry JB, Nelson SR, Samson FE, Pazdernik TL (1988b) Convulsions and cerebral inositol-1-phosphate levels in rats treated with diisopropyl fluorophosphate. Pharmacol Toxicol 63:137–138

Savolainen KM, Hirvonen M-R, Tarhanen J, Nelson SR, Samson FE, Pazdernik TL (1990) Changes in cerebral inositol-1-phosphate concentrations in LiCl-treated rats: regional and strain differences. Neurochem Res 15:541–545

Schreiber G, Avissar S, Aulakh CS, Murphy DL (1990) Lithium-selective alteration of the function of brain versus cardiac G_s protein. Neuropharmacology 29:1067–1071

Schreiber G, Avissar S, Danon A, Belmaker RH (1991) Hyperfunctional G proteins in mononuclear leukocytes of patients with mania. Biol Psychiatr 29:273–280

Schultz JE, Siggins GR, Schocker FW, Türck M, Bloom FE (1981) Effects of prolonged treatment with lithium and tricyclic antidepressants on discharge frequency, norepinephrine responses and beta receptor binding in rat cerebellum: electrophysiological and biochemical comparison. J Pharmacol Exp Ther 216:28–38

Sherman WR, Leavitt AL, Honchar MP, Hallcher LM, Phillips BE (1981) Evidence that lithium alters phosphoinositide metabolism: chronic administration elevates primarily D-myo-inositol-1-phosphate in cerebral cortex of the rat. J Neurochem 36:1947–1951

Sherman WR, Munsell LY, Gish BG, Honchar MP (1985) Effects of systemically administered lithium on phosphoinositide metabolism in rat brain, kidney, and testis. J Neurochem 44:798–807

Sherman WR, Gish BG, Honchar MP, Munsell LY (1986) Effects of lithium on phosphoinositide metabolism in vivo. Fed Proc 45:2639–2646

Sillence DJ, Downes CP (1992) Lithium treatment of affective disorders: effects of lithium on the inositol phospholipid and cyclic AMP signalling pathways. Biochim Biophys Acta 1138:46–52

Song L, Jope RS (1992) Chronic lithium treatment impairs phosphatidylinositol hydrolysis in membranes from rat brain regions. J Neurochem 58:2200–2206

Spiegel AM, Shenker A, Weinstein LS (1992) Receptor-effector coupling by G proteins: implications for normal and abnormal signal transduction. Endocr Rev 13:536–565

Staunton DA, Magistretti PJ, Shoemaker WJ, Deyo SN, Bloom FE (1982) Effects of chronic lithium treatment on dopamine receptors in the rat corpus striatum. II. No effect on denervation or neuroleptic-induced supersensitivity. Brain Res 232:401–412

Stubbs EB Jr, Agranoff BW (1993) Lithium enhances muscarinic receptor-stimulated CDP-diacylglycerol formation in inositol-depleted SK-N-SH neuroblastoma cells. J Neurochem 60:1292–1299

Takimoto K, Okada M, Matsuda Y, Nakagawa H (1985) Purification and properties of myo-inositol-1-phosphatase from rat brain. J Biochem 98:363–370

Türck M, Yeh H, Woodward DJ, Schultz JE (1981) β-Adrenergic receptors in rat cerebellum after neonatal X-irradiation: effect of prolonged imipramine and lithium treatment. Neurosci Lett 27:357–362

Volonté C (1988) Lithium stimulates the binding of GTP to the membranes of PC12 cells cultured with nerve growth factor. Neurosci Lett 87:127–132

Watanabe Y, Morita H, Imaizumi T, Takeda M, Hariguchi S, Nishimura T, Yoshida H (1990) Changes of ADP-ribosylation of GTP-binding protein by pertussis toxin in human platelets during long-term treatment of manic depression with lithium carbonate. Clin Exp Pharmacol Physiol 17:809–812

Watanabe Y, Kawamoto H, Imaizumi T, Sakagoshi N, Iwakura K, Morita H, Iwasaki T, Yoshida H (1991) Effects of lithium ion on the inhibitory GTP-binding protein and its coupling response. Cell Signal 3:59–64

Watson DG, Lenox RH (1996) Chronic lithium-induced down-regulation of MARCKS in immortalized hippocampal cells: potentiation by muscarinic receptor activation. J Neurochem 67:767–777

Weiner ED, Kalasapudi VD, Papolos DF, Lachman HM (1991) Lithium augments pilocarpine-induced fos gene expression in rat brain. Brain Res 553:117–122

Weiner ED, Mallat AM, Papolos DF, Lachman HM (1992) Acute lithium treatment enhances neuropeptide Y gene expression in rat hippocampus. Mol Brain Res 12:209–214

Whitworth P, Kendall DA (1988) Lithium selectively inhibits muscarinic receptor-stimulated inositol tetrakisphosphate accumulation in mouse cerebral cortex slices. J Neurochem 51:258–265

Whitworth P, Kendall DA (1989) Effects of lithium on inositol phospholipid hydrolysis and inhibition of dopamine D_1 receptor-mediated cyclic AMP formation by carbachol in rat brain slices. J Neurochem 53:536–541

Whitworth P, Heal DJ, Kendall DA (1990) The effects of acute and chronic lithium treatment on pilocarpine-stimulated phosphoinositide hydrolysis in mouse brain in vivo. Br J Pharmacol 101:39–44

Wolff J, Berens SC, Jones AB (1970) Inhibition of thyrotropin-stimulated adenyl cyclase activity of beef thyroid membranes by low concentration of lithium ion. Biochem Biophys Res Commun 39:77–82

Participation of Cytoskeletal Elements in Neuronal Signal Transduction: New Insight into the Molecular Basis of Antidepressant Action

SHINICHI HATTA and HIDEYO OHSHIKA

Introduction

Antidepressant drugs have been used clinically not only for depression but also for other psychiatric disorders. Despite extensive studies, the mechanisms of action of antidepressant drugs have not been clearly established. The classic monoamine hypothesis of depression suggests that depressive disorders are associated with subnormal monoamine release at certain synapses of the CNS. Antidepressant drugs are supposed to increase the availability of noradrenaline and serotonin, either by inhibiting amine reuptake or by blocking monoamine oxidase in presynaptic nerve terminals, and facilitate monoamine transmission (Schildkraut 1965). However, an acute effect of antidepressants on neurotransmission is inconsistent with the delayed onset of clinical efficacy of these drugs (Zemlan and Garver 1990). Furthermore, neuroleptic drugs such as amphetamine and cocaine that block reuptake or catabolism of monoamines do not have an antidepressant effect. Thus, an acute neurochemical effect of antidepressant drugs may not account for the mechanism of action of these drugs.

The most obvious biochemical effect of chronic treatment using antidepressant drugs is a reduction in sensitivity of β-adrenergic agonist-stimulated adenylyl cyclase (β-receptor desensitization), often paralleled by a decrease in the number of β-adrenergic receptors (down-regulation) (Sulser 1984). The mechanism of this receptor down-regulation is not yet clear; it may be secondary to the antidepressant-induced increase of neurotransmitters within the synaptic cleft. Although β-receptor changes occur with a delayed response, they still occur before the time required for clinical effects of antidepressants

Department of Pharmacology, School of Medicine, Sapporo Medical University, South-1, West-17, Chuo-ku, Sapporo, Hokkaido 060, Japan to develop. Furthermore, it is reported that β-receptor down-regulation is not related to the antidepressant effect (Chen and Rasenick 1995a). Thus, it is difficult to reconcile β-receptor down-regulation (loss of β-adrenergic stimulation to the neuron) with antidepressant effects.

It has been hypothesized that some biochemical or physiological changes in postreceptor components, including guanosine triphosphate (GTP)-binding proteins (G proteins) and adenylyl cyclase, may explain the common actions of antidepressant treatments (Menkes et al. 1983; Ozawa and Rasenick 1989). Studies in this and other laboratories have demonstrated that long-term treatment of rats with antidepressant drugs enhances 5′-guanylylimidodiphosphate (GppNHp)- or forskolin-stimulated adenylyl cyclase activity in brain membranes of rats (Newman and Lerer 1989; De Montis et al. 1990; Ozawa and Rasenick 1989, 1991; Chen and Rasenick 1995b). This effect correlates well with the time course of the clinical therapeutic response. It was also reported that GppNHp- or forskolin-stimulated adenylyl cyclase activity was reduced in brain membranes of depressed patients (Cowburn et al. 1994). These findings suggest that chronic treatment with antidepressant drugs enhances adenylyl cyclase activity, and this may be relevant to the therapeutic effects of antidepressants. However, the molecular basis of these antidepressant actions remains to be elucidated.

Recent evidence has suggested that antidepressants have a direct action on G proteins in vitro (Yamamoto et al. 1992; Ozawa et al. 1994). It might be possible, therefore, that altered postreceptor signal amplification after antidepressant treatment is due to a change in the amount or the function of G proteins. However, chronic treatment of rats with antidepressants promotes enhanced activation of adenylyl cyclase by Gs protein without changing the amount or the function of Gs protein (Ozawa and Rasenick 1989; Chen and Rasenick 1995b; Kamada et al. 1997). These findings support the idea that long-term antidepressant treatment results in the enhancement of coupling between Gs protein and the catalytic subunit of adenylyl cyclase rather than changing the quantity or quality of Gs protein itself in rat brain.

Chronic treatment with antidepressants may enhance the activation of Gs, consequently potentiating the activation of adenylyl cyclase through several intermediates. It is suggested that some membrane or cytoskeletal component is modified by chronic antidepressant treatment (Menkes et al. 1983). It is possible, therefore, that a modification of some membrane or cytoskeletal component induced by chronic antidepressant treatment contributes to enhanced coupling between Gs and adenylyl cyclase.

Tubulin, G Proteins, and Adenylyl Cyclase Signal Transduction

Microtubules are known to act as a structural element of the cell as well as participating in cell motility, mitosis, and axonal transport. In addition, several studies have suggested that microtubule elements act as modulators of the adenylyl cyclase signal transduction system (Zor 1983; Rasenick et al. 1985). Several early studies have demonstrated a potentiation of hormone-stimulated production of cyclic AMP with a decrease in microtubule polymerization by microtubule-disrupting drugs such as colchicine and vinblastine in leukocytes (Rudolph et al. 1979), lymphoma cells (Kennedy and Insel 1979), macrophages (Hagmann and Fishman 1980), and rat cerebral cortex synaptic membranes (Rasenick et al. 1981).

Tubulin, the primary constituent of microtubules, is a GTP-binding protein that shares many features with the signal-transducing G proteins. Tubulin consists of an $\alpha\beta$ heterodimer with a molecular weight of approximately 110kDa. Tubulin and adenylyl cyclase G proteins bind and hydrolyze GTP. Tubulin has at least two guanine nucleotide (GTP)-binding sites, one nonexchangeable at the α subunit, and the other exchangeable at the β subunit. Both tubulin and G proteins form complexes with other proteins, represented by microtubule assembly for tubulin and α, β, γ heterotrimer formation for G proteins, and the trigger for the formation and/or dissociation of the complex involves the exchange of guanosine diphosphate (GDP) for GTP. As in the case with G proteins, tubulin is also a substrate for pertussis- and cholera toxin-catalyzed ribosylation of ADP (Amir-Zaltsman et al. 1982; Lim et al. 1985). Considerable structural homology exists among a variety of G proteins, including those associated with adenylyl cyclase (Gs, Gi), the rod outer segment (Gt or transducin), protein synthesis (EFtu), and the *ras* oncogene product (p21). The similarities among G proteins evoke the possibility that tubulin, which is associated, perhaps intrinsically, with synaptic membranes (Zisapel et al. 1980; Stephens 1986), may interact with the adenylyl cyclase system in those membranes. Several recent studies indicate that one locus of interaction between cytoskeletal components and the adenylyl cyclase system is between tubulin and G proteins, which are known to be involved in the regulation of adenylyl cyclase.

Tubulin–G Protein Interaction

The G proteins, which are widely distributed, membrane-bound proteins, are involved in the coupling of numerous hormones and neurotransmitter receptors to their specific effectors in a large number of signal-transduction systems. The state of microtubule assembly as well as dimeric tubulin can modulate G-protein function. Recent studies have demonstrated that tubulin dimers specifically bind to and form a complex with the signal-transducing G proteins Gs and Gi_1 and, in the process of activating these proteins, modulate their functions (Wang et al. 1990). Tubulin modifies neuronal adenylyl cyclase signaling through the association of Gs and Gi, and a direct transfer of guanine nucleotide from the exchangeable GTP-binding site of tubulin to $Gs\alpha$ and $Gi\alpha$ is suggested as a mechanism of this regulation (Rasenick and Wang 1988).

In our previous studies (Hatta et al. 1994, 1995a,b), when rat cerebral cortex membranes were incubated with GppNHp-liganded tubulin (tubulin–

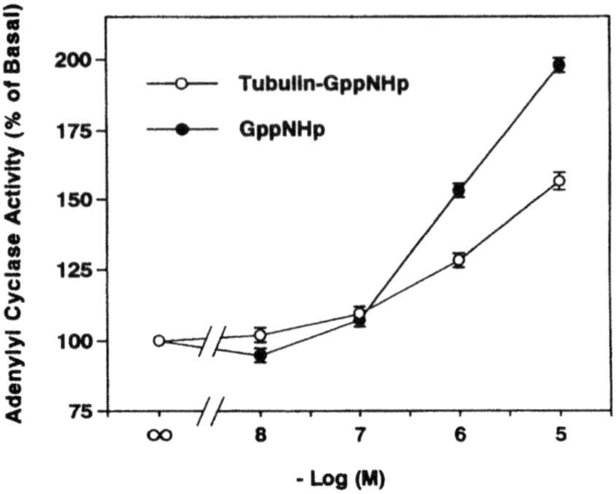

FIG. 1. Activation of adenylyl cyclase by tubulin–GppNHp and GppNHp in rat cerebral cortex synaptic membranes. Adenylyl cyclase activity was assayed under conditions optimal for stimulation of the enzyme [5 m*M* $MgCl_2$, 1 m*M* ethyleneglycoltetraacetic acid (EGTA) at 30°C] with the indicated concentrations of tubulin–GppNHp, prepared as described by Rasenick and Wang (1988), or GppNHp

GppNHp) and assayed for adenylyl cyclase under conditions optimal for stimulation of the enzyme, tubulin–GppNHp activated adenylyl cyclase, although the potency of tubulin–GppNHp was slightly lower than that of GppNHp (Fig. 1). On the other hand, under conditions in which inhibition rather than stimulation of adenylyl cyclase was favored, tubulin–GppNHp resulted in inhibition of the enzyme in a manner similar to that observed with GppNHp (Fig. 2). To examine whether guanine nucleotide could be transferred from tubulin to G proteins, tubulin was polymerized with the ^{32}P-labeled hydrolysis-resistant photoaffinity GTP analog, P^3-(4-azioanilido)-P^1-5′ GTP ([^{32}P]AAGTP). Addition of [^{32}P]AAGTP-liganded tubulin (tubulin–[^{32}P]AAGTP) to cortex membranes followed by a wash and UV photolysis resulted in the incorporation of AAGTP into Gsα and Giα, indicating transfer of AAGTP to Gsα and Giα from tubulin molecules (Fig. 3). These results further demonstrated that the tubulin dimer participates in the stimulatory and inhibitory regulation of adenylyl cyclase by transferring guanine nucleotide to Gsα and Giα, respectively.

In addition, it is noteworthy that, as a functional consequence of the interaction between tubulin and G proteins, tubulin can participate in the modulation of β-adrenergic, dopaminergic D_1 (Hatta et al. 1995a,b) and D_2 receptor function (Hatta et al. 1992). Furthermore, it was reported recently that tubulin activates Gq, which mediates activation of phospholipase $C\beta_1$, presumably through complex formation and nucleotide transfer between them, as in the case with Gs and Gi_1 (Popova et al. 1997).

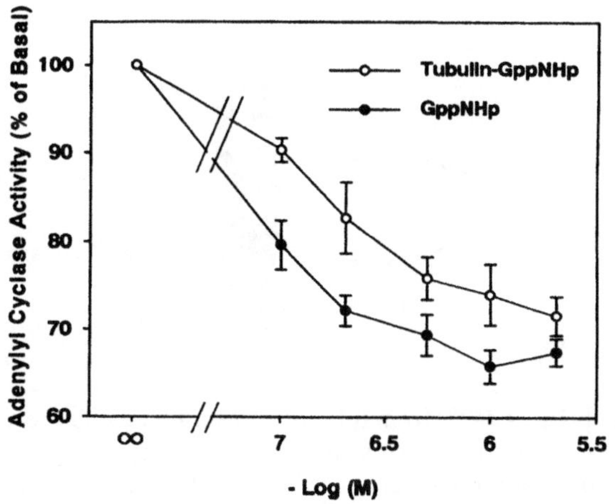

FIG. 2. Inhibition of adenylyl cyclase by tubulin-GppNHp and GppNHp in rat cerebral cortex synaptic membranes. Adenylyl cyclase activity was assayed under conditions in which inhibition rather than stimulation of adenylyl cyclase was favored (1 m*M* $MgCl_2$ at 23°C) with the indicated concentrations of tubulin–GppNHp, prepared as described by Rasenick and Wang (1988), or GppNHp

Tubulin–G protein complex formation occurs at regions of tubulin that are likely to be involved in binding of other tubulin dimers during the process of microtubule polymerization (Wang and Rasenick 1991). It has also been demonstrated that the formation of a complex between tubulin and Giα changes the GTP-binding characteristics of both molecules, and consequently, tubulin–Giα interaction stabilizes nucleotide binding in the complex (Roychowdhury et al. 1994). This may indicate that tubulin not only transfers nucleotides to G proteins, leading to their activation, but also stabilizes nucleotide binding through formation of a tubulin–G protein complex. Both guanine nucleotide transfer and the stabilization of the active Gα conformation lead to sustained activation of G protein by tubulin.

Tubulin represents a major component of the synaptic membrane (Bhattacharyya et al. 1985). Since microtubules have not been observed to associate with membranes (Stephens 1986), it is likely that much of this tubulin is present in dimer form. Recently, it has been demonstrated that in rat cerebral cortex postsynaptic densities, tubulin exists in preformed complexes with Gsα and $Gi_1α$ (Yan et al. 1996). Such complexes provide the physical framework for the interface between G protein-mediated signal transduction and the cytoskeleton. Interaction and complex formation between tubulin and G protein favorably occurs and, as a functional consequence of this, tubulin modulates adenylyl cyclase activity by transferring guanine nucleotide to Gs and Gi.

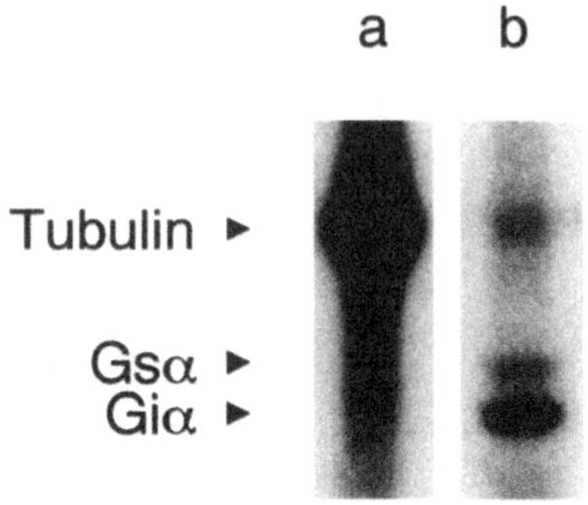

FIG. 3. Transfer of [^{32}P]AAGTP from tubulin to α subunits of G proteins in rat cerebral cortex membranes. Cerebral cortex membranes were incubated with 10 μg of [^{32}P]AAGTP-liganded tubulin (tubulin-[^{32}P]AAGTP) for 5 min (lane *b*). In lane *a*, 10 μg of tubulin-[^{32}P]AAGTP was UV-irradiated without incubating membranes. After incubation, the membranes were washed and subsequently subjected to photoaffinity labeling, sodium dodecyl sulfate-polyactylamide gel electrophoresis, and autoradiography. Addition of tubulin–[^{32}P]AAGTP to cortex membranes resulted in the incorporation of AAGTP into Gsα and Giα, with 4.7 ± 0.8% and 19.7 ± 1.2% of [^{32}P]AAGTP originally bound to tubulin, respectively. Incorporation of AAGTP into Gsα and Giα could be blocked by UV irradiation of tubulin–[^{32}P]AAGTP to covalently incorporate AAGTP into tubulin before incubation with cortex membranes, or by exposing the cortex membranes to an excess amount of GppNHp (10^{-4} *M*) to saturate the nucleotide-binding sites of the G protein before incubation with tubulin–[^{32}P]AAGTP (Hatta et al. 1994, 1995a). Similar results were obtained in rat striatal membranes (Hatta et al. 1995b)

Under physiological conditions, the guanine nucleotide that binds to the tubulin dimer is GTP. The hydrolysis of GTP by adenylyl cyclase-activating G proteins appears sufficiently slow (~0.2 mol Pi/mol Gi/min, and comparable GTPase activity for Gs) that transfer of GTP between tubulin and G proteins could occur within that time (Rasenick and Wang 1988). Thus, a population of GTP-loaded tubulin may provide a "GTP pool" for the activation of G proteins. The ability of the tubulin dimer to bind and transfer guanine nucleotide to Gs and Gi makes it a relevant candidate for an endogenous modulator of adenylyl cyclase.

Cytoskeletal Elements and Antidepressant Drugs

Several studies have demonstrated that long-term antidepressant treatment enhances guanine nucleotide-stimulated adenylyl cyclase in rat brain, suggesting that chronic antidepressant treatment alters some aspect of the membrane or cytoskeleton that promotes a more facile coupling between Gs and adenylyl

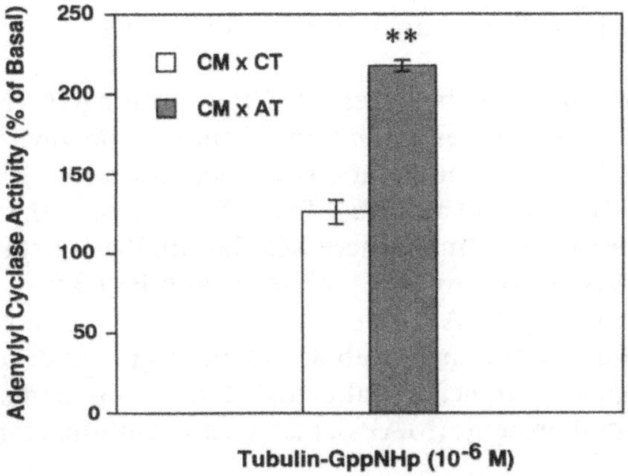

FIG. 4. Activation of adenylyl cyclase by tubulin–GppNHp prepared from control and amitriptyline-treated rats. Amitriptyline (10 mg/kg) was administered to male Sprague-Dawley rats by intraperitoneal injection once daily for 21 days, and control animals received saline as a vehicle. Rats were sacrificed 24 h after the final treatment, and cerebral cortex membranes or GppNHp-liganded tubulin was prepared. Adenylyl cyclase in cortex membranes prepared from control rats was assayed with 5 m*M* $MgCl_2$ and 1 m*M* EGTA at 30°C for 10 min in the presence of tubulin–GppNHp (10^{-6} *M*) prepared from control or amitriptyline-treated rats. The values are expressed as a percentage of the basal activity and shown as means ± SEM of six separate experiments. $^{**}P < 0.01$ indicates a significant difference compared with the activity of control tubulin in control cortex membranes. *CM × CT*, control membrane × control tubulin; *CM × AT*, control membrane × amitriptyline-treated tubulin

cyclase (Menkes et al. 1983; Ozawa and Rasenick 1989, 1991; Chen and Rasenick 1995b). Our recent findings support this idea (Kamada et al. 1997). As shown in Fig. 4, when tubulin–GppNHp prepared from chronically amitriptyline-treated rats (amitriptyline 10 mg/kg, i.p., once daily for 21 days) was incubated with cortex membranes prepared from control rats (CM × AT), the activation of adenylyl cyclase was significantly potentiated compared with that by tubulin–GppNHp prepared from the control (CM × CT). This result indicated that chronic treatment of the rat with amitriptyline altered the function of the tubulin dimer in a manner that resulted in enhancement of adenylyl cyclase activity. Since the protein levels of tubulin and G proteins (Gsα, Giα, Goα, Gqα, and Gβ) and the functions of Gs and Gi, estimated by immunoblotting and guanine nucleotide photoaffinity labeling with [^{32}P]AAGTP, respectively, were not changed by the treatment (Ozawa and Rasenick 1989; Kamada et al. 1997), it is suggested that long-term treatment with amitriptyline causes alterations in the functional interactions between tubulin and G proteins, and thereby the coupling of Gs to the catalytic subunit of adenylyl cyclase is enhanced. Thus, tubulin, a cytoskeletal element, is likely to be one of the intracellular target proteins for the actions of antidepressant drugs.

On the other hand, it has been reported that prolonged administration of antidepressants to rats causes inhibition of tubulin polymerization and an increase of phosphorylated microtubule-associated protein 2 (MAP_2) in the cerebral cortex (Miyamoto et al. 1995). These findings raise the possibility that chronic antidepressant treatment increases the number of tubulin dimers in the cerebral cortex. Furthermore, long-term antidepressant treatment has been shown to change cyclic AMP-dependent endogenous phosphorylation of MAP_2 in soluble and crude microtubule fractions (Perez et al. 1989). Thus, these findings appear to indicate that cytoskeletal components, including microtubule-associated proteins (MAPs), may be an additional target element of antidepressants.

MAPs are well established as important regulators of microtubule dynamics as well as contributors to the regulation of neuronal morphology and neurite outgrowth and regeneration, and they are considered a major structural component of the neuronal skeleton. MAP_2 binds to β-tubulin (Kim et al. 1986) near but not at a GTP-binding site (Littauer et al. 1985; Maccioni et al. 1985). The binding of MAP_2 to tubulin is regulated through phosphorylation of MAP_2, mediated by a cyclic AMP-dependent protein kinase (PKA) (Jameson et al. 1980) or Ca^{2+}/calmodulin-dependent protein kinase II (CaM-PK II) (Schulman 1984). Phosphorylation of MAP_2 results in a reduction of its binding to tubulin and inhibits tubulin polymerization (Jameson and Caplow 1981). Thus, microtubules may act not only as a component of the cytoskeleton, but also as a source of tubulin dimers, which, in turn, modify G-protein mediation of adenylyl cyclase. If antidepressant drugs inhibit the polymerization of tubulin by affecting cytoskeletal elements and, consequently, increasing the number of tubulin dimers, as has been suggested (Miyamoto et al. 1995), the increased tubulin dimers in synaptic membranes would associate more efficiently with the specific G proteins, leading to activation of G proteins via transfer of GTP from tubulin to α subunits of those G proteins. It is hypothesized that the mechanism of action of antidepressants may involve quantitative and qualitative modifications of tubulin molecules, which induce enhanced coupling between Gs and adenylyl cyclase catalytic molecules independently of β-adrenergic receptor down-regulation (Fig. 5).

Clearly, the above discussion is speculative, and much remains to be done before the molecular mechanism of antidepressant action affecting cytoskeletal components is understood. However, evidence that the targets of antidepressant drugs lie distal to neurotransmitter receptors has been accumulating. The presence of a well-organized network of cytoskeletal elements and the components of the G-protein-mediated neurotransmitter signal-transduction system may play an important role in the regulation of neurotransmitter responses (or responsiveness). Perhaps membrane tubulin serves to orchestrate intracellular responses to neurotransmitter signals. With

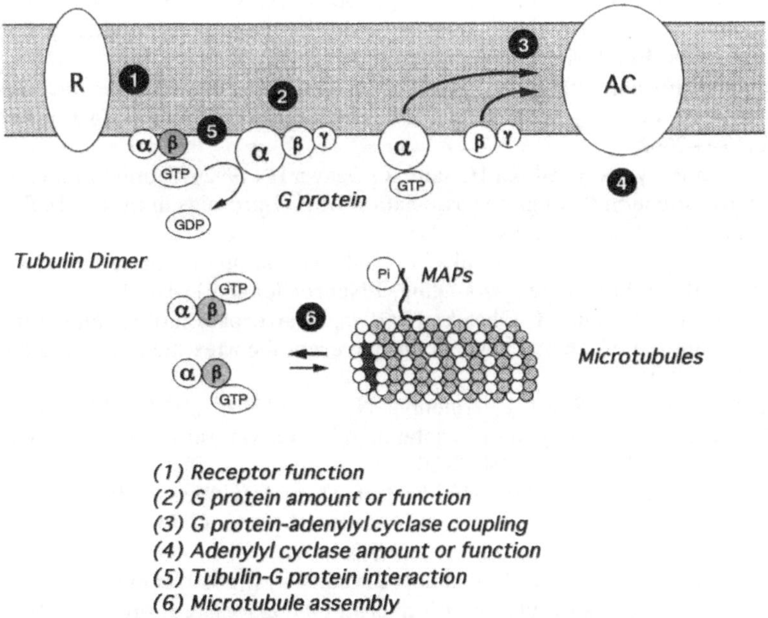

FIG. 5. Regulation of adenylyl cyclase and possible targets of antidepressant drugs. The figure depicts processes that might be altered as a result of chronic antidepressant treatment. *AC*, adenylyl cyclase; *GDP*, guanosine diphosphate; *GTP*, guanosine triphosphate; *R*, receptor; *MAPs*, microtubule-associated proteins

the addition of further information, it is hoped that a mechanistic understanding of the molecular basis of antidepressant action will be developed.

References

Amir-Zaltsman Y, Ezra E, Scherson T, Zutra A, Littauer UZ, Salomon Y (1982) ADP-ribosylation of microtubule proteins as catalyzed by cholera toxin. EMBO J 1:181–186

Bhattacharyya B, Sackett DL, Wolff J (1985) Tubulin, hybrid dimers and tubulin S: stepwise charge reduction and polymerization. J Biol Chem 260:10208–10216

Chen J, Rasenick MM (1995a) Chronic treatment of C6 glioma cells with antidepressant drugs increases functional coupling between a G protein (Gs) and adenylyl cyclase. J Neurochem 64:724–732

Chen J, Rasenick MM (1995b) Chronic antidepressant treatment facilitates G protein activation of adenylyl cyclase without altering G protein content. J Pharmacol Exp Ther 275:509–517

Cowburn RF, Marcusson JO, Eriksson A, Wiehager B, O'Neill C (1994) Adenylyl cyclase and G protein subunit levels in postmortem frontal cortex of suicide victims. Brain Res 633:297–304

De Montis GM, Devoto P, Gessa GL, Procella A, Serra G, Tagliamonte A (1990) Selective adenylate cyclase increase in the limbic area of long-term imipramine-treated rats. Eur J Pharamcol 180:169–174

Hagmann J, Fishman PH (1980) Modulation of adenylate cyclase in intact macrophage by microtubules: opposing actions of colchicine and chemotactic factor. J Biol Chem 255:2659–2662

Hatta S, Ameniya N, Ohshika H, Saito T, Ozawa H (1992) Tubulin modifies neuronal sinal transduction through the association with G-proteins in rat cerebral cortex and striatum. Soc Neurosci Abstr 18:285

Hatta S, Ozawa H, Saito T, Ohshika H (1994) Alteration of tubulin-Gi protein interaction in rat cerebral cortex with aging. J Neurochem 63:1104–1110

Hatta S, Ozawa H, Saito T, Ohshika H (1995a) Participation of tubulin in the stimulatory regulation of adenylyl cyclase in rat cerebral cortex membranes. J Neurochem 64:1343–1350

Hatta S, Ozawa H, Saito T, Ameniya N, Ohshika H (1995b) Tubulin stimulates adenylyl cyclase activity in rat striatal membranes via transfer of guanine nucleotide to Gs protein. Brain Res 704:23–30

Jameson L, Caplow M (1981) Modification of microtubule steady-state dynamics by phosphorylation of the microtubule-associated proteins. Proc Natl Acad Sci USA 78:3413–3417

Jameson L, Frey T, Zeeberg B, Dalldorf F, Caplow M (1980) Inhibition of microtubule assembly by phosphorylation of microtubule-associated proteins. Biochemistry 19:2472–2479

Kamada H, Ozawa H, Saito T, Hatta S, Takahata N (1997) Dimeric tubulin-stimulated adenylyl cyclase activity is augmented after long-term amitriptyline treatment. Life Sci 60:57–66

Kennedy MS, Insel PA (1979) Inhibitors of microtubule assembly enhance beta-adrenergic and prostaglandin E_1-stimulated cyclic accumulation in S49 lymphoma cells. Mol Pharmacol 16:215–223

Kim H, Jensen C, Rebhun L (1986) The binding of MAP-2 and tau on brain microtubules in vitro: implications for microtubule structure. Ann NY Acad Sci 466:218–239

Lim L-K, Sekura RD, Kaslow HR (1985) Adenine nucleotides directly stimulate pertussis toxin. J Biol Chem 260:2585–2588

Littauer U, Giveon D, Thierauf M, Ginsburg I, Postingl H (1985) Tubulin binding sites for microtubule associated proteins. In: De Brabander M, De Mey J (eds) Microtubules and microtubule inhibitors 1985. Elsevier Science Publishers B.V., Amsterdam, pp 171–176

Maccioni R, Serrono L, Avila J (1985) Structural and functional domains of tubulin. BioEssays 4:165–169

Menkes DB, Rasenick MM, Wheeler MA, Bitensky NW (1983) Guanosine triphosphate activation of brain adenylate cyclase: enhancement by long-term antidepressant treatment. Science 219:65–67

Miyamoto S, Asakura M, Sasuga Y (1995) Effect of chronic administration of antidepressants on microtubule assembly in rat cerebral cortex. Jpn J Psychopharmacol 15:385–395 (abstract in English)

Newman ME, Lerer B (1989) Post-mediated increases in adenylate cyclase activity after chronic antidepressant treatment: relationship to receptor desensitization. Eur J Pharmacol 162:345–352

Ozawa H, Rasenick MM (1989) Coupling of the stimulatory GTP-binding protein Gs to rat synaptic membrane adenylate cyclase is enhanced subsequent to chronic antidepressant treatment. Mol Pharmacol 36:803–808

Ozawa H, Rasenick MM (1991) Chronic electroconvulsive treatment augments coupling of the GTP-binding protein Gs to the catalytic moiety of adenylyl cyclase in a manner similar to that seen with chronic antidepressant drugs. J Neurochem 56:330–338

Ozawa H, Katamura Y, Hatta S, Amemiya N, Saito T, Ohshika H, Takahata N (1994) Antidepressants directly influence in situ binding of guanine nucleotide in synaptic membrane. Life Sci 54:925–932

Perez J, Tinelli D, Brunello N, Racagni G (1989) cAMP-dependent phosphorylation of soluble and crude microtubule fractions of rat cerebral cortex after prolonged desmethylimipramine treatment. Eur J Pharmacol Mol Pharmacol Sec 172:305–316

Popova JS, Garrison JC, Rhee SG, Rasenick MM (1997) Tubulin, Gq, and phosphatidylinositol 4,5-bisphosphate interact to regulate phospholipase Cβ_1 signaling. J Biol Chem 272:6760–6765

Rasenick MM, Wang N (1988) Exchange of guanine nucleotides between tubulin and GTP-binding proteins that regulate adenylate cyclase: cytoskeletal modification of neuronal signal transduction. J Neurchem 51:300–311

Rasenick MM, Stein P, Bitensky MW (1981) The regulatory subunit of adenylate cyclase interacts with cytoskeletal components. Nature 294:560–562

Rasenick MM, O'Callahan CM, Moore CA, Kaplan RS (1985) GTP-binding proteins which regulate neuronal adenylate cyclase interact with microtubule proteins. In: De Brabander M, De Mey J (eds) Microtubules and microtubule inhibitors 1985. Elsevier Science Publishers B.V., Amsterdam, pp 313–323

Roychowdhury S, Wang N, Rasenick MM (1994) Tubulin-G protein association stabilizes GTP binding and activates GTPase: cytoskeletal participation in neuronal signal transduction. Biochemistry 33:9800–9805

Rudolph SA, Hegstrand LR, Greengard P, Malawista SE (1979) The interaction of colchicine with hormone-sensitive adenylate cyclase in human leukocytes. Mol Pharmacol 16:805–812

Schildkraut JJ (1965) The catecholamine hypothesis of affective disorders: a review of supporting evidence. Am J Psychiatry 122:509–522

Schulman H (1984) Differential phosphorylation of MAP-2 stimulated by calcium-calmodulin and cyclic AMP. Mol Cell Biol 4:1175–1178

Stephens RE (1986) Membrane tubulin. Biol Cell 57:95–110

Sulser F (1984) Antidepressant treatments and regulation of norepinephrine-receptor-coupled adenylate cyclase systems in brain. Adv Biochem Psychopharmacol 39:249–261

Wang N, Rasenick MM (1991) Tubulin-G protein interactions involve microtubule polymerization domains. Biochemistry 30:10957–10965

Wang N, Yan K, Rasenick MM (1990) Tubulin binds specifically to the signal-transducing proteins, Gsα and Giα_1. J Biol Chem 265:1239-1242.

Yamamoto H, Tomita U, Mikuni M, Kobayasi I, Kagaya A, Katada T, Ui M, Takahashi K (1992) Direct activation of purified Go-type GTP binding protein by tricyclic antidepressants. Neurorosci Lett 139:194–196

Yan K, Greene E, Belga F, Rasenick MM (1996) Synaptic membrane G proteins are complexed with tubulin in situ. J Neurochem 66:1489–1495

Zemlan FP, Garver DL (1990) Depression and antidepressant therapy: receptor dynamics. Prog Neuropsychopharmacol Biol Psychiatry 14:503–523
Zisapel N, Levi M, Gozes I (1980) Tubulin: an integral protein of mammalian synaptic vesicle membranes. J Neurochem 34:26–32
Zor U (1983) Role of cytoskeletal organization in the regulation of adenylate cyclase-cyclic adenosine monophosphate by hormones. Endocr Rev 4:1–21

In Vivo Investigations of Signal-Transduction Systems in Affective Disorders by Magnetic Resonance Spectroscopy

TADAFUMI KATO

Introduction

In vivo nuclear magnetic resonance spectroscopy (MRS) is a noninvasive tool that can detect various molecules at around millimolar concentrations in living human organs. The nuclei of many species of atoms, such as ^{1}H, ^{7}Li, and ^{31}P, have magnetic properties and can be used for in vivo MRS. Because the principles of MRS are complicated and not easily summarized, only a brief introduction is given here. For details, see other review articles (Nasrallah and Pettegrew 1995; Kato et al. in press).

When the radio frequency (RF) pulse of a particular frequency (Larmor frequency) is applied to a nuclear spin under a static magnetic field, the nuclear spin resonates and absorbs energy. When the nuclear spin then returns to the previous state, it emits electromagnetic waves. This emission is known as free induction decay (FID), and the overall process is referred to as relaxation. The concentration of nuclei is related to the intensity of FID observed. Generally, many FIDs must be averaged to obtain enough signal for quantitative analysis. Because the Larmor frequency changes not only with the type of nuclei but also with the type of chemical bonding with other nuclei, the small difference in resonance frequency dependent on the position of the nuclei in a molecule, the chemical shift, enables us to discriminate different molecules containing the same nuclei. Many kinds of signal localization methods have been used to obtain MR signals from regions of the brain. To obtain MR spectra from FID or echoes, several data-processing techniques should be applied.

Department of Neuropsychiatry, Faculty of Medicine, University of Tokyo, 7-3-1 Hongo, Bunkyo-ku, Tokyo 113, Japan

Which Metabolites in Signal-Transduction Systems Can Be Measured by MRS?

Neurotransmitters

The concentrations of neurotransmitters such as dopamine, noradrenaline, and serotonin are too small (around $10 \mu M$) to be analyzed by MRS. Nor can MRS discriminate signals of acetylcholine from those of other molecules containing trimethylamine residues, such as free choline, phosphocholine (PCho), glycerophosphocholine (GPC), and phosphatidylcholine (PtdCho), which exist at much concentrations.

The most promising application of MRS for the study of neurotransmitters is the detection of amino acids, such as glutamate and γ-amino butyric acid (GABA), that can be observed by ^{1}H-MRS. These signals are complicated by strong J-couplings and are difficult to resolve from nearby signals with conventional ^{1}H-MRS spectra (Fig. 1). GABA (Petroff et al. 1995) and glutamate (Crozier et al. 1990) can be detected by ^{1}H-MRS with high resolution by the use of spectral editing techniques. It has also been reported that glutamate/glutamine (Glx) resonance can be clearly seen at a lower magnetic field (0.5T) than usual (1.5T) (Prost et al. 1997).

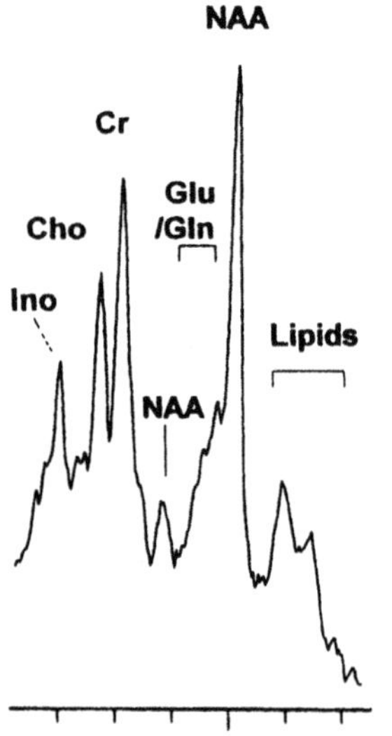

FIG. 1. Proton magnetic resonance spectrum in the left basal ganglia detected by the stimulated echo method (STEAM) in a normal control subject. Echo time is 20 ms. *Ino*, *myo*-inositol; *Cho*, choline-containing compounds; *Cr*, creatine and phosphocreatine; *NAA*, *N*-acetylaspartate; *Glu/Gln*, glutamate/glutamine

It should be noted that the concentration of molecules detectable by ^1H-MRS may not reflect neurotransmitter activity but rather a pool of these metabolites. In spite of this limitation, determining the concentration of neurotransmitters by ^1H-MRS has clinical significance under certain conditions. Petroff et al. (1995) examined the concentration of GABA by spectral editing technique and found that it markedly increased during treatment with vigabatrin, which inhibits GABA transaminase. On the other hand, levels of GABA were decreased in the brain in patients with alcoholism (Behar et al. 1996). The concentration of Glx increased in the brain in patients with hepatic encephalopathy (Kleis et al. 1992). An increase of Glx in these patients was correlated with psychiatric symptoms caused by hepatic encephalopathy (Bayer et al. 1996). Although it was reported that glutamate levels were significantly lower and glutamine levels significantly higher in the frontal cortex in nontreated schizophrenic patients than in normal controls (Stanley et al. 1995), this finding has yet to be reproduced. It should be noted that contamination of protein signals makes it difficult to examine glutamate and glutamine separately.

A more direct approach for quantitating the dynamics of glutamate is the heteronuclear multiquantum coherence (HMQC) method. With this technique, ^{13}C nuclei are irradiated by an RF pulse with a frequency of ^{13}C, transferred from ^{13}C to ^1H, and detected by a proton coil with a higher sensitivity than that used in the detection of ^{13}C itself. Although this method involves the application of expensive ^{13}C-glucose, it can detect kinetic parameters of glutamate synthesis with high spatial resolution (Inubushi et al. 1993). The technique could be applied to clinical studies and is superior to positron emission tomography (PET) for examining glutamate synthesis because it can discriminate metabolites such as glucose, glutamate, and lactate by a difference of chemical shift, whereas PET cannot resolve all molecules containing the radiolabeled carbon. This method enables us to examine the time course of glutamate synthesis in vivo.

Second Messengers

The application of MRS to the study of second-messenger systems is even more promising, because the effect of a neurotransmitter is amplified at the second-messenger level and large biochemical reactions can be elicited with small numbers of neurotransmitter molecules.

Phosphoinositide System

Stimulation of receptors by agonists, such as acetylcholine or serotonin, causes hydrolysis of phosphatidylinositol bisphosphate (PIP_2) via activation of phospholipase C (PLC) by receptor-coupled guanosine triphosphate (GTP)-binding protein (Fig. 2). PIP_2 is metabolized to form diacylglycerol (DG) and inositol triphosphate (IP_3). DG activates protein kinase C (PKC). PKC phos-

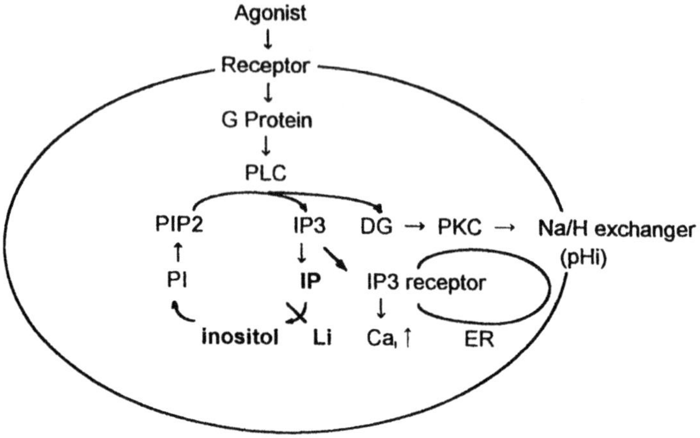

FIG. 2. Phosphoinositide second-messenger system. *DG*, diacylglycerol; *ER*, endoplasmic reticulum; *IP*, inositol-1-phosphate; *IP3*, inositol triphosphate; *pH$_i$*, intracellular pH; *PI*, phosphatidylinositol; *PIP2*, phosphatidylinositol diphosphate; *PKC*, protein kinase C; *PLC*, phospholipase C

phorylates many kinds of proteins to modulate cellular functions, including the sodium proton (Na^+/H^+) exchanger, which mediates intracellular pH (pH_i). On the other hand, IP_3 binds to IP_3 receptor on the surface of the endoplasmic reticulum, which results in an increase of intracellular calcium ($[Ca]_i$). An increase of $[Ca]_i$ causes various cellular responses. IP_3 is metabolized to form inositol-1-phosphate (I1P), and I1P is broken down into *myo*-inositol by inositol-1-phosphatase. Lithium is reported to strongly inhibit this enzyme, and I1P accumulates in the brain at concentrations on the order of millimolar during lithium treatment. This causes an intracellular deficiency of *myo*-inositol, because *myo*-inositol cannot be transported from the extracellular compartment. An intracellular deficiency of *myo*-inositol causes the inactivation of phosphoinositide signal-transduction systems. This mechanism is the most commonly accepted hypothesis of the clinical action of lithium (see El-Mallakh 1996 for review).

In this pathway, several metabolites can be measured by MRS. Renshaw et al. (1986) first applied ^{31}P-MRS to investigate the phosphoinositide signal-transduction system. They examined brain ^{31}P-MR spectra in cats receiving lithium chloride systemically. After lithium treatment, the phosphomonoester (PME) peak was increased. When the brain was extracted and examined by in vitro nuclear magnetic resonance (NMR), the increase in the PME peak was found to be caused by an increase in I1P. They also found that the PME peak was increased after cholinergic stimulation by pilocarpine treatment during chronic treatment with lithium (Renshaw et al. 1987). These results were reproduced by Preece et al. (1992). Silverstone et al. (1996) were the first to apply this technique to humans. They found that lithium treatment alone did not increase the PME peak detected by ^{31}P-MRS in normal volunteers. In a subsequent study, however, they found that the PME peak was increased after amphetamine challenge during chronic treatment with lithium in normal volunteers (Silverstone, personal communication).

The concentration of *myo*-inositol can also be examined by ^{1}H-MRS. Therefore, it was expected that the inositol deficiency hypothesis for lithium could be tested using ^{1}H-MRS. However this signal, termed the "inositol peak", is actually contaminated with I1P (Cerdan et al. 1986). Therefore, a decrease in *myo*-inositol from lithium treatment would be compensated by an increase in I1P. In fact, the "inositol peak" detected by in vivo ^{1}H-MRS was not decreased in rat brain (Preece et al. 1992), in the brains of patients with bipolar disorder (Bruhn et al. 1993), or in the brains of normal volunteers (Silverstone et al. 1996) during chronic lithium treatment. On the other hand, *myo*-inositol detected by in vitro high-resolution ^{1}H-NMR was decreased in brain extracts from rats treated with lithium (Preece et al. 1992).

It is of note that the concentration of lithium can also be examined by ^{7}Li-MRS in vivo (Kato et al. 1994). If ^{31}P- and ^{7}Li-MRS are combined, the activity of the phosphoinositide signaling system should be measurable in living human brains. Mikuni et al. (1991) examined serotonin-induced accumulation of I1P in platelets incubated with lithium and found that it was enhanced in patients with affective disorders compared with controls. A similar experiment could be done in the human brain using in vivo ^{31}P- and ^{7}Li-MRS in clinical settings. It has been postulated that the phosphatidylinositol (PI) signaling system is impaired in patients with bipolar disorder (Soares and Mallinger 1996). Direct assessment of the phosphoinositide second-messenger system by ^{31}P- and ^{7}Li-MRS should resolve this ambiguity.

Intracellular pH increases during agonist stimulation via activation of the Na^+/H^+ exchanger. An agonist-dependent increase in pH_i was also detected by ^{31}P-MRS in vitro (Podo et al. 1987). Sappey-Marinier et al. (1992a) first reported that pH_i tended to be increased in the visual cortex during photic stimulation in normal volunteers. This finding was confirmed in our study (Kato et al. 1996a). The increase in pH_i may be caused by agonist-dependent activation of the Na^+/H^+ exchanger, though further studies are needed to clarify the biochemical characteristics of this phenomenon.

Other Phospholipases

Phospholipase D (PLD) is a signal-transduction system that has recently drawn attention (Fig. 3). The enzyme is known to be coupled to the stimulation of metabotropic glutamate receptor, endothelin ETB receptor, and histamine H_1 receptor. The pathway may be mediated at least partly by a GTP-binding protein. PLD hydrolyzes PtdCho to form phosphatidic acid (PA) and free choline (Cho). Although the activity of this enzyme is usually quantitated by the formation of PA or phosphatidylethanol in vitro, an increase in choline may also reflect the activity of this signal-transduction system

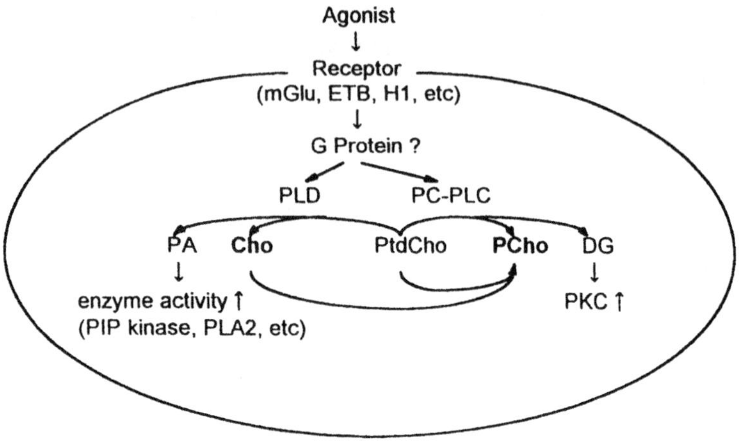

FIG. 3. Phospholipase D signal-transduction system. *Cho*, choline; *DG*, diacylglycerol; *ETB*, endothelin B receptor; *H1*, histamine 1 receptor; *mGlu*, metabotropic glutamate receptor; *PA*, phosphatidic acid; *PC-PLC*, phosphatidylcholine-selective phospholipase C; *PtdCho*, phosphatidylcholine; *PCho*, phosphocholine; *PIP*, phosphatidylinositol; *PLA2*, phospholipase A2; *PLD*, phospholipase D; *PKC*, protein kinase C

under certain experimental conditions. It was reported that Cho accumulates in the brain during energy deprivation due to aglycemia, anoxia, and ischemia, and this was ascribed to the activation of PLD (Djuricic et al. 1991).

PtdCho-selective phospholipase C (PC-PLC) also hydrolyzes PtdCho to form PCho and DG.

Activation of phospholipase A_2 (PLA_2) causes hydrolysis of PtdCho to form lyso-PtdCho and free fatty acids. Lyso-PtdCho is rapidly broken down into glycerophosphocholine (GPC), PCho, and Cho.

The Cho peak detected by ^{1}H-MRS contains Cho, PCho, and GPC; the PME peak detected by ^{31}P-MRS contains PCho; and the phosphodiester (PDE) peak detected by ^{31}P-MRS contains GPC and PtdCho. Therefore, under certain experimental conditions, alteration of these metabolites by activation of a particular phospholipase may be detectable by ^{1}H- and ^{31}P-MRS.

Li et al. (1993) examined the human visual cortex with proton-decoupled ^{31}P-MRS and found that GPC and glycerophosphoethanolamine (GPE) concentrations were significantly decreased during photic stimulation. The biochemical background of this phenomenon is also of interest.

Cyclic AMP

The concentration of intracellular cyclic AMP (cAMP) is on the order of micromolar, which is much smaller than that of ATP (millimolar). Therefore, cAMP usually cannot be detected by ^{31}P-MRS under physiological conditions.

However, when the breakdown of cAMP was inhibited by a phosphodiesterase inhibitor, 3-isobutyl-1-methylxanthine (IBMX), cAMP became detectable by ^{31}P-MRS during stimulation by melanocyte-stimulating hormone (MSH) and forskolin in melanoma cells (Degani et al. 1991) or β-adrenergic stimulation by isoproterenol in C6 glioma cells (Pianet et al. 1992). Cyclic AMP may be detectable by ^{31}P-MRS in the human brain after agonist stimulation during chronic treatment with the phosphodiesterase inhibitor, loripram. If so, it will provide a promising strategy to assess the in vivo activity of cAMP signal-transduction systems in the brain in patients with affective disorders.

Experiments with melanocytes (Degani et al. 1991) and C6 glioma cells (Pianet et al. 1992) unexpectedly revealed that phosphoethanolamine (PEt) levels increased during agonist stimulation of the cells. These results suggest that there is an unknown signal-transduction system mediated by hydrolysis of phosphatidylethanolamine generating PEt, which is known to act as a cholinergic enhancing factor (Bostwick et al. 1989).

Clinical Applications of MRS to the Study of Signal-Transduction Systems

In most clinical MRS studies, MR spectra were obtained at rest, without any activation. Therefore, even if the concentration of a certain metabolite in a signal-transduction system is higher or lower than that in normal controls, it is difficult to draw a definite conclusion as to how signal-transduction systems are impaired. As discussed above, a specific experimental design is needed to examine the activity of certain signal-transduction systems in vivo.

Phosphoinositide System

We used ^{31}P-MRS to examine whether I1P accumulated in the brain in patients with bipolar disorder who were treated with lithium (Kato et al. 1991). We examined phosphorus metabolism in the frontal lobes of 11 patients with bipolar disorder and 11 age-matched normal controls using the DRESS (depth-resolved surface coil spectroscopy) method. Nine of these patients were examined in the manic state and nine in the euthymic state. All were treated with lithium carbonate, and most of the manic patients were treated with additional antipsychotic drugs. We found a significant increase in the PME peak in the manic state compared with controls. Although the nine euthymic patients were also treated with lithium, the PME peak in these patients was not increased compared with that in controls (Fig. 4). In one patient, the time course of the PME peak was examined. Before the initiation of lithium treatment, the PME peak was normal. One week after the initiation of lithium treatment, the peak maximized, gradually decreasing thereafter. We postulated that this difference was due to an increase of I1P, and that the state-

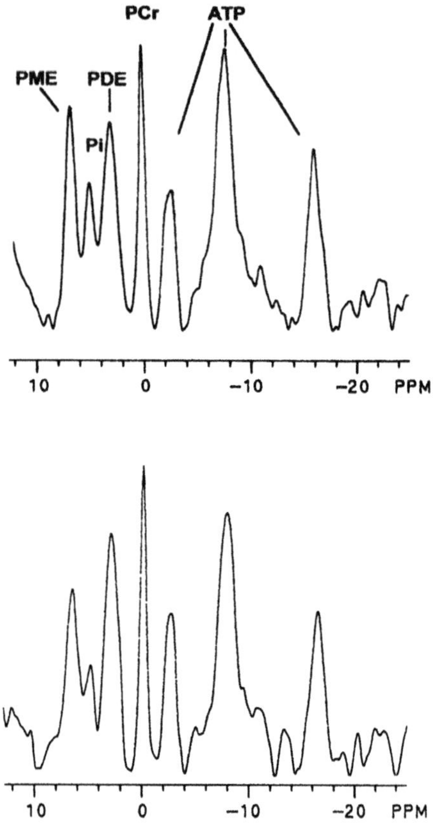

FIG. 4. Phosphorus-31 magnetic resonance spectra recorded in the frontal lobes in a patient with bipolar disorder (18 years old, male) treated with lithium in the manic state (*upper*) and in the euthymic state (*lower*). The upper spectrum was recorded 53 days after the initiation of lithium treatment. At that time, the lithium concentration was 0.6 m*M* in serum and 0.3 m*M* in brain. The lower spectrum was recorded 41 days after the upper, and the lithium concentration was 0.5 m*M* in serum and 0.4 m*M* in brain. On both occasions, no additional drug was administered. The PME peak area ratio dropped remarkably from 14.0% (*upper*) to 11.0% (*lower*). *PCr*, phosphocreatine; *PDE*, phosphodiester; *Pi*, inorganic phosphate; *PME*, phosphomonoester

dependent increase in I1P was due to a state-dependent alteration of phosphoinositide turnover in bipolar disorder.

There are many factors to consider when interpreting these results, notably, the effects of a state-dependent alteration of lithium concentration in the brain, the duration of lithium treatment, the contribution of other metabolites in the PME region, and the effects of antipsychotic medication.

First, using ^{7}Li-MRS, we examined whether lithium concentrations in the brain change with mental state in patients with bipolar disorder. We found a patient whose lithium concentration rapidly increased, exceeding the concentration in serum at the time of the manic switch, and returned to prior levels after the manic switch (Kato et al. 1992). However, there was no significant difference between manic and euthymic patients in the ratio of brain to serum lithium (Kato et al. 1992). Lithium concentrations in the brain and serum were not correlated in the manic state but were significantly correlated in the euthymic and depressive states (Kato et al. 1994). Although the effects of a state-dependent alteration of lithium concentration in the brain cannot be completely excluded, as noted above, such effects are unlikely, because there was no significant correlation between brain lithium concentration and PME in patients with bipolar disorder (Kato et al. 1993).

Next, the effects of the duration of lithium treatment were examined. The PME peak ratio was significantly higher in manic patients treated with lithium for less than 2 weeks than in those treated for more than 2 weeks (Kato in press). This is compatible with the finding by Renshaw et al. (1987) that the PME peak maximized 1 week after the initiation of lithium treatment and decreased thereafter. There was a discrepancy between our first report (Kato et al. 1991), in which the PME peak was higher in 9 manic patients than in 11 normal controls, and our second study (Kato et al. 1993), in which there was no significant difference between 17 manic patients and 17 controls in the PME peak. Differences in the duration of lithium treatment might have confounded these results, as the duration of treatment was longer in the second study.

In our study, control subjects did not receive lithium, which complicated the interpretation of the results. Silverstone et al. (1996) reported that the PME peak did not increase during 1 week of lithium treatment in human volunteers. The lithium concentration in serum and the duration of lithium treatment did not differ from that in our manic patients who showed an increase in the PME peak. On the other hand, Silverstone et al. (unpublished) found that the PME peak increased in humans given amphetamine after long-term treatment with lithium. These results are compatible with the hypothesis that phosphoinositide turnover via monoaminergic stimulation is increased in manic patients.

Using ^{31}P-MRS, Keshavan et al. (1995) examined the effects of lithium on drug-free patients with schizophrenia. They did not find an increase in the PME peak 1 week after initiation of treatment. This, together with the finding by Silverstone et al. (1996), suggests that the increase in PME during lithium treatment is specific to mania. In our study of schizophrenia, the PME peak did not differ between drug-free patients and patients treated with antipsychotic drugs (Kato et al. 1995).

These findings are compatible with our first hypothesis that the phosphoinositide pathway is increased in the frontal lobes of patients with bipolar disorder in the manic state. However, the following questions remain to be clarified: Is the increase in the PME peak state-dependent or trait-dependent? Is the increase in the PME peak actually due to an increase of

I1P? Is this finding due to hyperactivity of monoaminergic neurons or a hypersensitivity to neurotransmitters in patients with bipolar disorder?

Recently, the development of a technique of proton-decoupled ^{31}P-MRS made it possible to discriminate PEt from PCho in the PME peak. I1P may be resolved from PEt and PCho and quantitatively analyzed by this sophisticated MRS technique, although it has never been reported to date. In our study, we examined manic patients at different intervals after the initiation of lithium treatment with uncontrolled medication. Examination of more consistent intervals and the administration of amphetamine or related substances should provide evidence of increased phosphoinositide metabolism.

As noted above, pH_i is partly regulated by the phosphoinositide signal-transduction system. We found that pH_i was lower in euthymic patients with bipolar disorder treated with lithium than in controls, whereas it was increased in the manic state (Kato et al. 1993). We hypothesized that this is due to increased phosphoinositide turnover. However, several factors need to be taken into consideration before drawing a definite conclusion.

Choline

Choline-containing compounds detected by ^{1}H-MRS in the basal ganglia were present in significantly higher concentrations in patients with major depression (Charles et al. 1994; Renshaw et al. 1994) and bipolar disorder (Kato et al. 1996b) than in controls. This may be due to increased activation of phospholipases, as noted above. Christensen et al. (1994) found that the PDE peak detected by ^{31}P-MRS was increased in the basal ganglia in medicated patients with major depression and hypothesized that the increases in the Cho peak by ^{1}H-MRS and the PDE peak by ^{31}P-MRS in the basal ganglia are due to an increase in GPC. However, the PDE peak was normal in a subsequent study in drug-free patients with major depression (Moore et al. 1997). Therefore, the increase in the Cho peak in drug-free patients with major depression may be due to an increase in free choline. The Cho peak detected by ^{1}H-MRS was higher in the white matter hyperintensity lesion (WMHI) delineated by T_2-weighted MRI (Sappey-Marinier et al. 1992b). It is a relatively consistent finding that WMHIs occur frequently in patients with affective disorders. The finding that PLD-induced accumulation of free Cho in the brain during ischemia suggests that the increase in the Cho peak in the subcortical region in patients with major depression and bipolar disorder is caused by increased activity of PLD due to ischemia. However, it is difficult to conclude from these results that a certain phospholipase is activated during major depression, because several other factors affect the concentrations of Cho-containing compounds in the brain.

The Cho peak was increased after ingestion of 50 mg/kg Cho, but this uptake decreased with age (Cohen et al. 1995). It was also reported that the increase in the Cho peak after ingestion of Cho was associated with a better response to Cho augmentation for lithium therapy of rapid-cycling bipolar disorder (Stoll et al. 1996). These results suggest a role of Cho transport function in bipolar disorder.

Lipids

Using ^{1}H-MRS, Woods and Ciu (1990) found that the lipid peak was significantly elevated after electroconvulsive therapy. They speculated that this increase was due to an increase in free fatty acids and DG caused by hydrolysis of inositol phospholipids (Ciu and Woods 1995). Although this finding was not confirmed in humans (Felber et al. 1993) or in animals (Prichard et al. 1987), submillimolar concentrations of free fatty acids on DG would theoretically be detectable by ^{1}H-MRS. However, it should be noted that signals from lipids participating in signal-transduction systems can easily be contaminated by signals from fat outside the volume of interest.

Conclusion

Several signal-transduction systems, such as the inositol phospholipid pathway, phospholipase D or other phospholipases, and cAMP, can be examined in living human brain by using ^{31}P-, ^{1}H-, and ^{7}Li-MRS. Amino acid neurotransmitters such as glutamate and GABA can be examined by ^{1}H-MRS. To date, clinical MRS studies suggest that the phosphoinositide signaling pathway is activated in mania. A well-organized study design using MRS and a pharmacological activation in clinical settings is needed for in vivo assessment of signal-transduction systems in affective disorders.

Acknowledgments. The author is grateful to all who contributed to the study project, particularly Jun Murashita, M.D., Hiroshi Hamakawa, M.D., and Toshiro Inubushi, Ph.D. The author also thanks Saburo Takahashi, M.D., Ph.D., and Nobumasa Kato, M.D., Ph.D., for continued support.

References

Bayer S, Laubenberger J, Haussinger D, Hennig J, Langer M (1996) Correlation of cerebral metabolites with clinical findings in hepatic encephalopathy observed by ^{1}H-MRS (abstract). Proceedings of the International Society of Magnetic Resonance in Medicine (ISMRM), Berkeley, 412

Behar K, Rothman D, Petersen K, Hooten M, Namanworth S, Petroff OAC, Shulman G, White J, Petrakis I, Charney D, Krystal J (1996) Cortical GABA levels are reduced in localized ^{1}H-NMR spectra of alcoholic and hepatic encephalopathy patients. Proceedings of the International Society of Magnetic Resonance in Medicine, Berkeley, 408

Bostwick JR, Landers DW, Craford G, Lau K, Appel SH (1989) Purification and characterization of a central cholinergic enhancing factor from rat brain: its identity as phosphoethanolamine. J Neurochem 53:448–458

Bruhn H, Stoppe G, Staedt J, Merboldt KD, Hänicke W, Frahm J (1993) Quantitative proton MRS in vivo shows cerebral myo-inositol and cholines to be unchanged in manic-depressive patients treated with lithium (abstract). Proceedings of the Society of Magnetic Resonance in Medicine, Berkeley, 1543

Cerdan S, Hansen CA, Johannsen R, Inubushi T, Williamson JR (1986) Nuclear magnetic resonance spectroscopic analysis of myo-inositol phosphates including inositol 1,3,4,5-tetrakisphosphate. J Biol Chem 261:14676–14680

Charles HC, Lazeyras F, Krishnan KRR, Boyko OB, Payne M, Moore D (1994) Brain choline in depression: in vivo detection of potential pharmacodynamic effects of antidepressant therapy using hydrogen localized spectroscopy. Prog Neuro-Psychopharmacol Biol Psychiatry 18:1121–1127

Chiu TM, Woods BT (1995) MRS and levels of free fatty acid in brain after electroconvulsive therapy. In: Nasrallah HA, Pettegrew JW (eds) NMR spectroscopy in psychiatric brain disorders. American Psychiatric Press, Washington, DC, pp 235–252

Christensen JD, Renshaw PF, Stoll AL, Lafer B, Fava M (1994) ^{31}P-spectroscopy of the basal ganglia in major depression (abstract). Proceedings of Society of Magnetic Resonance in Medicine, Berkeley, 608

Cohen BM, Renshaw PF, Stoll AL, Wortman RJ, Yorgelun-Todd D, Babb SM (1995) Decreased brain choline uptake in older adults. An in vivo proton magnetic resonance spectroscopy study. JAMA 274:902–907

Crozier S, Brereton IM, Rose SE, Field J, Shannon GF, Doddrell DM (1990) Application of volume-selected, two-dimensional multiple-quantum editing in vivo to observe cerebral metabolities. Magn Reson Med 16:496–502

Degani H, DeJordy JO, Salomon Y (1991) Stimulation of cAMP and phosphomonoester production by melanotropin in melanoma cells: ^{31}P-NMR studies. Proc Natl Acad Sci USA 88:1506–1510

Djuricic B, Olson SR, Assaf HM, Whittingham TS, Lust WD, Drewes LR (1991) Formation of free choline in brain tissue during in vitro energy deprivation. J Cereb Blood Flow Metab 11:308–313

El-Mallakh RS (1996) Lithium. Actions and mechanisms. American Psychiatric Press, Washington, DC

Felber SR, Pycha R, Hummer M, Aichner FT, Fleischhacker WW (1993) Localized proton and phosphorus magnetic resonance spectroscopy following electroconvulsive therapy. Biol Psychiatry 33:651–654

Inubushi T, Morikawa S, Kito K, Arai T (1993) ^{1}H-detected in vivo ^{13}C-NMR spectroscopy and imaging at 2T magnetic field: efficient monitoring of ^{13}C-labeled metabolites in the rat brain derived from 1-^{13}C-glucose. Biochem Biophys Res Commun 191:866–872

Kato T, Shioiri T, Takahashi S, Inubushi T (1991) Measurement of phosphoinositide metabolism in bipolar patients using in vivo ^{31}P-MRS. J Affect Disord 22:185–190

Kato T, Takahashi S, Inubushi T (1992) Brain lithium concentrations by ^{7}Li and ^{1}H magnetic resonance spectroscopy in bipolar disorder. Psychiatry Res Neuroimaging 45:53–63

Kato T, Takahashi S, Shioiri T, Inubushi T (1993) Alterations in brain phosphorus metabolism in bipolar disorder detected by in vivo ^{31}P and ^{7}Li magnetic resonance spectroscopy. J Affect Disord 27:53–60

Kato T, Takahashi S, Inubushi T (1994) Brain lithium concentration measured with lithium-7 magnetic resonance spectroscopy: A review. Lithium 5:75–81

Kato T, Shioiri T, Murashita J, Hamakawa H, Takahashi Y, Inubushi T, Takahashi S (1995) Lateralized abnormality of high energy phosphate and bilateral reduction of phosphomonoester measured by ^{31}P-MRS of the frontal lobes in schizophrenia. Psychiatry Res Neuroimaging 61:151–160

Kato T, Murashita J, Shioiri T, Hamakawa H, Inubushi T (1996a) Effect of photic stimulation on energy metabolism in the human brain measured by ^{31}P-MR spectroscopy. J Neuropsychiatry Clin Neurosci 8:417–422

Kato T, Hamakawa H, Shioiri T, Murashita J, Takahashi Y, Takahashi S, Inubushi T (1996b) Choline-containing compounds detected by proton magnetic resonance spectroscopy in the basal ganglia in bipolar disorder. J Psychiatry Neurosci 21:248–254

Kato T, Inubushi T, Kato N (in press) Magnetic resonance spectroscopy in affective disorders. J Neuropsychiatry Clin Neurosci

Keshavan MS, Pettegrew JW, Panchlingam K (1995) MRS in the study of psychoses: psychopharmacological studies. In: Nasrallah HA, Pettegrew JW (eds) NMR spectroscopy in psychiatric brain disorders. American Psychiatric Press, Washington, DC, pp 131–146

Kleis R, Ross BD, Farrow NA, Ackerman Z (1992) Metabolic disorders of the brain in chronic hepatic encephalopathy detected with H-1 MR spectroscopy. Radiology 182:19–27

Li SJ, Prost RW, Tan SG, Charles HC (1993) The decrease in phosphodiesters during photic stimulation in human primary visual cortex. Proceedings of the Society of Magnetic Resonance in Medicine, 65

Mikuni M, Kusumi I, Kagaya A, Kuroda Y, Mori H, Takahashi K (1991) Increased 5HT-2 receptor function as measured by serotonin-stimulated phosphoinositide hydrolysis in platelets of depressed patients. Prog Neuropsychopharmacol Biol Psychiatry 15:49–61

Moore CM, Christensen JD, Lafer B, Fava M, Renshaw PF (1997) Lower levels of nucleoside triphosphate in the basal ganglia of depressed subjects: a phosphorus-31 magnetic resonance spectroscopy study. Am J Psychiatry 154:116–118

Nasrallah HA, Pettegrew JW (eds) (1995) NMR spectroscopy in psychiatric brain disorders. American Psychiatric Press, Washington, DC

Petroff OAC, Rothman DL, Behar KL, Mattson RH (1995) Initial observations on effect of vigabatrin on in vivo ^{1}H spectroscopic measurements of γ-aminobutyric acid, glutamate, glutamine in human brain. Epilepsia 36:457–464

Pianet I, Canioni P, Labouesse J, Merle M (1992) β-Adrenergic stimulation of C6 glioma cells: effects of cAMP overproduction on cellular metabolites. A multinuclear NMR study. Eur J Biochem 209:707–715

Podo F, Carpinelli G, DiVito M, Giannini M, Proietti E, Fiers W, Gresser L, Belardelli F (1987) Nuclear magnetic resonance analysis of tumor necrosis factor-induced alterations of phospholipid metabolites and pH in Friend leukemia cell tumors and fibrosarcomas in mice. Cancer Res 47:6481–6489

Preece NE, Gadian DG, Houseman J, Williams SR (1992) Lithium-induced modulation of cerebral inositol phosphate metabolism in the rat. A multinuclear magnetic resonance study in vivo. Lithium 3:287–297

Prichard JW, Petroff OAC, Ogino T, Shulman RG (1987) Cerebral lactate elevation by electroshock: a ^{1}H magnetic resonance study. Ann NY Acad Sci 508:54–63

Prost RW, Mark L, Mewissen M, Li SJ (1997) Detection of glutamate/glutamine resonances by ^{1}H magnetic resonance spectroscopy at 0.5 Tesla. Magn Reson Med 37:615–618

Renshaw PF, Summers JJ, Renshaw CE, Hines KG, Leigh JS Jr (1986) Changes in the P-31 NMR spectra of cats receiving lithium chloride systemically. Biol Psychiatry 21:694–698

Renshaw PF, Schnall MD, Leigh JS Jr (1987) In vivo P-31 NMR spectroscopy of agonist-stimulated phosphatidylinositol metabolism in cat brain. Magn Reson Med 4:221–226

Renshaw PF, Lafer B, Christensen JD, Stoll AL, Rothschild A, Fava M, Rosenbaum JF, Cohen BM (1994) Proton MRS of the basal ganglia in major depression (abstract). Biol Psychiatry 35:685

Sappey-Marinier D, Calabrese G, Fein G, Hugg JW, Biggins C, Weiner MW (1992a) Effect of photic stimulation on human visual cortex lactate and phosphates using ^{1}H and ^{31}P magnetic resonance spectroscopy. J Cereb Blood Flow Metab 12:584–592

Sappey-Marinier D, Calabrese G, Hetherington HP, Fisher SN, Deicken R, VanDyke C, Fein G, Weiner MW (1992b) Proton magnetic resonance spectroscopy of human brain: applications to normal white matter, chronic infarction, and MR imaging white matter signal hyperintensities. Magn Reson Med 26:313–327

Silverstone PH, Hanstock CC, Fabian J, Staab R, Allen PS (1996) Chronic lithium does not alter human myo-inositol or phosphomonoester concentrations as measured by ^{1}H- and ^{31}P-MRS. Biol Psychiatry 40:235–246

Soares JC, Mallinger AG (1996) Abnormal phosphatidylinositol (PI)-signaling in bipolar disorder. Biol Psychiatry 39:461–462

Stanley JA, Drost DJ, Williamson PC, Carr TJ (1995) In vivo proton MRS study of glutamate and schizophrenia. In: Nasrallah HA, Pettegrew JW (eds) NMR spectroscopy in psychiatric brain disorders. American Psychiatric Press, Washington DC, pp 21–44

Stoll AL, Sachs GS, Cohen BM, Lafer B, Christensen JD, Renshaw PF (1996) Choline in the treatment of rapid-cycling bipolar disorder: clinical and neurochemical findings in lithium-treated patients. Biol Psychiatry 40:382–388

Woods BT, Chiu TM (1990) In vivo ^{1}H spectroscopy of the human brain following electroconvulsive therapy. Ann Neurol 28:745–749

GPSR Compliance

The European Union's (EU) General Product Safety Regulation (GPSR) is a set of rules that requires consumer products to be safe and our obligations to ensure this.

If you have any concerns about our products, you can contact us on ProductSafety@springernature.com

In case Publisher is established outside the EU, the EU authorized representative is:

Springer Nature Customer Service Center GmbH
Europaplatz 3
69115 Heidelberg, Germany

Batch number: 10844692

Printed by Printforce, the Netherlands